# THE ESSENTIAL GUIDE TO CHILDREN'S VACCINES

## Books in the Healthy Home Library Series
## from St. Martin's Paperbacks

# THE ESSENTIAL GUIDE TO CHILDREN'S VACCINES

Deborah Mitchell

A Lynn Sonberg Book

St. Martin's Paperbacks

Notice: This book is intended as a reference volume only, not as a medical manual. The information given here is designed to help you make informed decisions about your health. It is not intended as a substitute for any treatment that may have been prescribed by your doctor. If you suspect that you have a medical problem, we urge you to seek competent medical help.

Mention of specific companies, organizations, or authorities in this book does not imply endorsement by the author or publisher, nor does mention of specific companies, organizations, or authorities imply that they endorse this book, its author or the publisher.

Internet addresses given in this book were accurate at the time it went to press.

THE ESSENTIAL GUIDE TO CHILDREN'S VACCINES

Copyright © 2012 by Lynn Sonberg.

All rights reserved.

For information address St. Martin's Press, 175 Fifth Avenue, New York, NY 10010.

EAN: 978-1-250-00219-8

Printed in the United States of America

St. Martin's Paperbacks edition / November 2012

St. Martin's Paperbacks are published by St. Martin's Press, 175 Fifth Avenue, New York, NY 10010.

10  9  8  7  6  5  4  3  2  1

# CONTENTS

# INTRODUCTION

One of the most important decisions you will ever make as a parent regarding your children's health concerns vaccinations. From the moment your child is born, you are faced with a decision about the first vaccine on the list of childhood vaccinations recommended by the Centers for Disease Control and Prevention (CDC)—the vaccine for hepatitis B—and you will be asked to make many more decisions about this and other vaccines throughout your child's young and adolescent life.

Before the introduction of vaccines, parents did not have these decisions to make, but then millions of children and adults contracted, suffered, and died of diseases that today we consider to be completely or largely preventable. One of the diseases that comes to mind is smallpox, which was one of the deadliest scourges known to humans, killing an estimated 300 million or more people during the twentieth century alone. Thus far it is the only disease affecting humans that has been eradicated by vaccination, with the last known case appearing in Somalia in 1977.

Vaccines also are responsible for controlling many infectious diseases that were once significantly more common in the United States, especially among children, including polio, measles, mumps, diphtheria, whooping cough (pertussis), German measles (rubella), and tetanus. According to a report by researchers at the Pediatric Academic Society, childhood vaccinations in the United States prevent about 10.5 million cases of infectious illness and thirty-three thousand deaths per year.[1] In short, vaccinations could arguably be said to be one of the greatest medical discoveries of all time.

One example of the importance of vaccines was illustrated recently. In December 2010, health experts and leaders from around the world made a commitment to dedicate the next ten years to the Decade of Vaccines. Their hope and goal is to pursue research into the development and delivery of vaccines to people around the world, especially children in the poorest countries. This effort will be funded by governments and the private sector, including the Bill & Melinda Gates Foundation, which committed $10 billion over the decade.[2]

But are vaccines safe? More and more parents and health experts are questioning whether the standard regimen of vaccines for infants, children, and adolescents is entirely safe, especially as the number of recommended vaccines continues to grow.

An illustration of some of the concerns parents have about vaccines can be seen in a June 2011 report from *Health Affairs,* in which federal health researchers questioned parents about vaccinations. Although nearly 95 percent of parents said they would vaccinate their children, more than three-quarters expressed concern about a wide range of immunization issues, such as the number of recommended injections, side effects of the vaccinations, and possible complications such as autism and other health issues. The study's authors emphasized that parents need to have reliable sources of information as they contemplate the risks and benefits of vaccinating their children and whether they will indeed get the recommended immunizations.

I hope *Essential Guide to Children's Vaccines* will provide you with information to help you make decisions about the vaccinations that have been recommended and mandated for your children. This book contains the latest available information culled from a variety of reliable sources and presents it in an easy-to-access format.

Vaccines and vaccinations are a hot topic and sometimes a controversial and confusing one. That's why it can help to have a reliable source to turn to for unbiased information so you can make your own choices. This book is such a source.

## WHY THIS BOOK IS IMPORTANT

Vaccinating your child is a decision you as a parent should make **only** after you have reviewed what is known thus far about each type of vaccination and the disease it is designed to prevent. After all, every disease for which there is a vaccine is not the same: they differ in how likely it is your child will get the disease, the complications associated with the disease, the seriousness of the consequences of not getting vaccinated, and the side effects associated with the vaccine.

The information gathered together for *Essential Guide to Children's Vaccines* came from experts and institutions in both mainstream and complementary medicine; for example, the U.S. Public Health Service's Advisory Committee on Immunization Practices (ACIP), the Centers for Disease Control and Prevention (CDC), the American Academy of Pediatrics Committee on Infectious Diseases, the Holistic Pediatric Association, ProCon.org, ThinkTwice Global Vaccine Institute, and experts such as Dr. Stephanie Cave, Dr. Paul A. Offit, Dr. Kenneth Bock, and Dr. Robert Sears, among others. In essence, this book has done much of the detective work for you. But that does not mean your job is done; I have just provided you with information and tools to facilitate your journey.

## HOW TO USE THIS BOOK

The first chapter introduces you to how vaccines work—what they are, the different types, and how they impact an infant's immune system. Chapter 2 addresses a topic on every parent's mind: vaccine safety. Here is where I discuss concerns about whether too many vaccines are given at one time, if additives and preservatives in vaccines are safe, and whether vaccines are given at too young an age.

The next twelve chapters of the book are arranged in the same order in which the Centers for Disease Control and Prevention recommends children's vaccines be given, beginning with the hepatitis B vaccine at birth and ending with the vaccines recommended up to age 18. The twelve recommended vaccines are, in this order:

- Hepatitis B

- Rotavirus

- Diphtheria/tetanus/pertussis

- *Haemophilus influenza* type B

- Pneumococcal disease

- Influenza

- Measles/mumps/rubella (MMR)

- Chicken pox (varicella)

- Polio

- Hepatitis A

- Meningococcal disease

- Human papillomavirus (HPV)

Naturally, because several vaccinations are recommended within the same general time frame, readers should not take the order of the chapters to mean they are to follow it

**exactly:** the decisions about vaccination schedules are made between parents and doctors. This book facilitates the process by including information about each vaccine as well as provides charts on when each vaccine is recommended to be given, including a catch-up chart that includes suggested times for vaccines children may have missed.

Each chapter on a vaccine discusses:

- the disease for which the vaccine is given, including its signs and symptoms, causes, treatments, and complications

- the recommended age(s) for administering the vaccine

- what the vaccine is made of

- reported side effects

- who should not get the vaccine

- who manufactures the vaccine

- controversies surrounding the vaccine

Whenever appropriate or relevant, the results of scientific research are also included.

The individual vaccine chapters are followed by the chapter "Action Plan: How to Individualize Your Child's Vaccination Schedule," which provides information on options available for parents who do not want to give one or more vaccines to their children (including information on alternative schedules), what to do if your child experiences an adverse reaction to a vaccine, the Vaccine Injury Compensation Program, and how to find the right pediatrician. The final chapter discusses vaccines for keeping your children safe when they travel outside of the United States.

In the appendices, I discuss getting help with the cost of

vaccines, provide the Centers for Disease Control and Prevention's schedules of vaccinations for children 0 to 6 years and 7 to 18 years and the catch-up schedule, and provide a list of Web sites that approach the issue of children's vaccinations from both sides of the controversy.

As a parent, you naturally want to do what is best for your children when it comes to their health. To make those critical and often hard decisions, you need unbiased information that presents both sides of the issue. Then, combining this information with professional advice, you can make an educated, informed decision. This book is a tool to help with that decision process.

# CHAPTER 1

How Vaccines Work

What are vaccines? How do they work? These are two seemingly simple questions, but the answers can't be given in a neat sound bite. So, I'm going to ask you to join me for several moments to learn some basic but important information about vaccines.

## WHAT ARE VACCINES?

The use of vaccines is based on a simple premise: it is better to prevent a disease than to treat it. Vaccines are substances that prevent disease in the individuals who receive them and protect people who have contact with others who have not been vaccinated.

Basically, vaccines work like this: A weakened or dead form of the organism—typically a bacterium or virus—that causes a specific disease is injected into the body. In the case of combination vaccines, the injection contains weakened forms of more than one organism. The body then produces substances called antibodies to fight the invading organisms, thereby developing immunity against the disease. Those antibodies remain in the body, so if the individual ever has contact with the disease-causing germs the antibodies will be there to destroy them and thus ward off illness.

The main purpose of a vaccine is to stimulate the body to form a high enough concentration of antibodies so that individuals can continue to be protected against the disease. As long as you keep your antibody concentration high (also known as titers, or blood immunity levels), you should have immunity. Vaccinating your child against any specific disease is not a 100 percent guarantee he or she will not get the disease or experience some mild symptoms. However, in most cases, the vaccine provides adequate protection against the disease. That is not to say vaccines do not also cause side effects or complications; they can and do, and this is a topic discussed throughout the book.

## HISTORY OF VACCINES IN A NUTSHELL

In the late eighteenth century, Edward Jenner discovered that if he inoculated people with the animal disease called cowpox, people would become immune to the human disease smallpox. Then, in 1885, Louis Pasteur worked on a method called attenuation, which is the use of a weakened form of a virus to provide immunity. As you will see in the following chapters, attenuated vaccines are still widely used today.

Vaccines really burst onto the U.S. scene with the discoveries made by Jonas Salk and Albert Sabin, both of whom developed a vaccine for polio. Salk is credited with an injectable vaccine that was first administered in 1955, while Sabin developed a live oral vaccine in 1961, which was later discontinued in the United States, but an injectable polio vaccine is still used today.

The childhood vaccines parents are familiar with today are the result of years of experimentation, evolution, and development. The first measles vaccine was licensed in 1963, and in the years that followed other childhood vaccines now recommended by the Advisory Committee on Immunization Practices to the Centers of Disease Control and Prevention became part of the current vaccination schedules. And the story is not over: new vaccines, new combinations and formulations, and new dosing recommendations are being announced all the time.

## AN INFANT'S IMMUNE SYSTEM

An infant's immune system does not kick into gear until the child is about 6 months old. During those first six months, children depend on the antibodies they received from their mother through the placenta during pregnancy. The only antibodies that cross the placenta are immunoglobulin G (IgG), which makes up 75 to 80 percent of all the antibodies in the body. Mothers who breast-feed their infants continue to pass these essential antibodies plus others via breast milk, which contains five types of antibodies, immunoglobulin A, D, E, G, and M. These antibodies provide a great deal of protection for infants, but they are not foolproof, and so infants are still vulnerable to numerous infectious diseases, such as whooping cough.

### Passive Immunity

The type of immunity infants receive from their mothers is called passive immunity because the mother passes her antibiotics to her child. During the first several months of an infant's life, the levels of the antibodies passed from the mother decline steadily. Fortunately, a healthy baby's immune system will begin to produce its own antibodies by age 2 to 3 months. Production is slow at the beginning, however, and so antibodies are not made at a normal rate until about age 6 months in healthy infants.

Please note that I am talking about "healthy" babies, so infants who have a chronic medical condition or who have an infection or other health issue may not reach a normal rate of antibody production until later. This is a concern you will need to discuss with your health-care provider.

When infants are injected with vaccines, they receive the same antigens or parts of antigens that cause disease. However, the antigens in the vaccines have been either killed or greatly weakened (attenuated) (I discuss these types of vaccine later), which means although they are not potent enough to cause symptoms or the disease, they are strong enough to stimulate production of antibodies. Therefore, when children are vaccinated they can develop immunity without having to experience the actual diseases the vaccines are designed to prevent.

### Another Type of Passive Immunity

Another type of passive immunity is called herd immunity. This means that an individual who has not been vaccinated at all or has been only partially vaccinated (e.g., has received only part of a necessary series of doses to achieve full immunity) may be protected against getting the disease if all or most of the people around him or her have been vaccinated. That is, the "herd" provides some protection for individuals who have not developed immunity.

Occasions when herd immunity is important include when a very young infant (younger than 6 or 8 weeks old) may be in close contact with other children or adults who have not been vaccinated and when a child who has not been vaccinated attends school with other children who have received their vaccinations. (Read more about herd immunity in chapter 2.)

## TYPES OF VACCINES

I have already mentioned the two basic forms of vaccines: killed (also known as inactivated or dead) and live. There is a third type, recombinant DNA vaccine, which is the newest member of the vaccine family and the result of genetic engineering. Here are the basics on each of the three types of vaccines.

## Killed Vaccines

To make a killed vaccine, the disease-causing organisms are deactivated, which means, unlike live vaccines, they cannot reproduce nor can they cause the disease they were created to prevent. Because the organisms have been killed, they trigger a weaker response by the immune system than do live vaccines. For this reason they also tend to be safer than live vaccines for certain populations, including pregnant women, children younger than 12 months, and anyone who has a compromised immune system.

As you will learn when you read about different killed vaccines, which are used for hepatitis A, hepatitis B, flu, pertussis, polio (injected), rabies, and typhoid, these vaccines are protein based, like the bacteria they mimic. Some of these bacteria have sugars called polysaccharides on their surface. When scientists created pure polysaccharide vaccines, they discovered these vaccine were not effective in infants. However, when the scientists combined (conjugated) the polysaccharide to a protein they were able to develop vaccines that were effective for infants and young children.

Another type of killed vaccine is a toxoid, which is made when scientists deactivate the poisons (toxins) that are produced by bacteria and viruses responsible for certain diseases. The vaccines to help prevent diphtheria and tetanus are toxoids. You can read more details about toxoids in chapter 5.

## Live Vaccines

To create a live vaccine, scientists use the living microorganisms (usually viruses) that cause the disease in question. The viruses are attenuated, or weakened, so they will not cause the disease, but at the same time they will stimulate the body's immune system to create an immune response. Examples of live attenuated viral vaccines include those for measles, mumps, chicken pox (varicella), rubella, and yellow fever. Live bacterial vaccines include one for typhoid fever and one for tuberculosis (Bacillus Calmette-Guérin vaccine).

## Recombinant DNA Vaccines

A third type of vaccine is a recombinant DNA vaccine, which is genetically engineered. To make a recombinant vaccine, scientists take specific genes from the infectious agent (e.g., virus, bacteria) and add them to a culture medium, such as yeast or a special broth. The hepatitis B vaccine is an example of a recombinant DNA vaccine, because it is made by culturing a part of the hepatitis B virus gene—the hepatitis B surface antigen (HBsAg)—in baker's yeast.

# CHAPTER 2

## Vaccines: Are They Safe?

*How safe are the vaccines recommended for my children?*
This is a question on the minds of the majority of parents.
When it comes to vaccine safety, the most common concerns expressed by parents are:

- How safe are the ingredients in my child's vaccines?

- Do doctors give too many vaccines and too soon?

- Does the MMR vaccine increase the risk of autism?

These questions do not have simple "yes" or "no" answers,
and well-informed experts have differing opinions about
them.

There are two other safety-related concerns that trouble
parents. One is the right of parents to refuse vaccines for
their children. Vaccinations are recommended by the federal government but mandated by individual states. In every
state, parents have at least one way to opt out of vaccinations
for their child. Because this is also an issue concerning personal choice, I discuss this question in depth in chapter 15,
on how to individualize your child's vaccination program.

The other safety-related issue is also a moral one of the public good versus the rights of the individual. For example, if you do decide to exercise your right not to have your child vaccinated, he or she could transmit disease to a vulnerable child who might be seriously harmed. Some physicians feel so strongly about the importance of universal vaccinations that they refuse care to children whose parents will not let their kids be vaccinated. Because this is an issue that parents should consider when they are choosing a pediatrician for their child, I discuss it in chapter 15, in the section "Finding the Right Pediatrician."

My goal in this chapter is to present a brief summary of the latest opinions and knowledge about vaccine safety. Because vaccine research is ongoing, I encourage you to ask your own questions of a trusted health-care provider and to keep up with the latest information on vaccine safety as it becomes available in the press and through your physician.

## HOW SAFE ARE THE INGREDIENTS IN MY CHILD'S VACCINES?

Just like the packaged foods you buy at the grocery store, your child's vaccines have an ingredient list, yet many parents never see it. In this book I reveal the production ingredients and additives found in children's vaccines. There is no doubt that some of the ingredients in vaccines are toxic. Few people can argue with the fact that formaldehyde and ethylene glycol (antifreeze) are substances you do not want to give your children. For children who have allergies to certain substances, such as latex or eggs, vaccines that have these ingredients can pose a danger as well.

However, the debate is over whether the small amounts of these ingredients present in vaccines are sufficient to cause adverse and/or long-lasting effects to the body, brain, or both. While the Food and Drug Administration (FDA), CDC, and vaccine manufacturers say the amounts of toxins in vaccines are insignificant and harmless, some experts disagree. Parents have the right to know what is in the vaccines so they can make an informed decision about whether the products are safe for their children.

Basically, there are four different types of substances involved in the vaccine production process:

- Vaccine production media (the material in which the vaccine components are cultured)

- Suspending fluid (e.g., saline, sterile water, or fluids that contain protein)

- Excipients (preservatives and stabilizers)

- Adjuvants or enhancers

Which of these substances are in your child's vaccines? The answer is not always simple, because each vaccine contains different ingredients. To help you identify what's in your child's vaccines, I tell you what is in each vaccine discussed in this book and the amount, which you will find in their respective chapters. You can get additional information about individual ingredients in the glossary, and the World Association for Vaccine Education (WAVE) is also an excellent source of information. (See the appendices.)

In addition, there are two vaccine additives that are of particular concern to parents—thimerosal and aluminum—and so I cover them in detail here.

## Thimerosal

Thimerosal is a mercury-containing organic compound (nearly 50 percent mercury by weight) that has been used in various drug products, including vaccines, since the 1930s. It is added to these produces to help prevent potentially life-threatening contamination with harmful organisms. In recent years, thimerosal became a very controversial topic in the vaccine world because it was being added to vaccines administered to children and because mercury is a neurotoxin (damages brain cells).

In July 1999, the American Academy of Pediatrics, the Public Health Service agencies, and vaccine makers agreed that thimerosal should be eliminated or reduced in vaccines as a precautionary measure. Therefore, thimerosal has been removed or is present in only trace amounts in all vaccines that are recommended for children ages 6 years of age and younger, with the exception of inactivated flu vaccine. (See the "Thimerosal in Vaccines" table.) A limited supply of preservative-free inactivated flu vaccine (which contains trace amounts of thimerosal) is available for infants, children, and pregnant women.

Much of the concern about thimerosal in vaccines involves its potential link with autism. In a study conducted by the Centers for Disease Control and Prevention and published in *Pediatrics* in October 2010, titled "Prenatal and Infant Exposure to Thimerosal from Vaccines and Immunoglobins and Risk of Autism," investigators reported there was no increased risk of autism associated with prenatal and early-life exposure to ethylmercury from vaccines or immunoglobulin preparations that contain thimerosal.

They based their conclusions on an analysis of 1,008 children, 256 of whom had autism spectrum disorder and 752 who did not. After the researchers identified exposure to ethylmercury from thimerosal in the children and their mothers, they found that children who had any type of autism spectrum disorder and the children who were free of any such disorder had had similar exposure to ethylmercury from pregnancy to age 20 months. The researchers then concluded that thimerosal-containing immunizations did not increase the risk of autism spectrum disorders.

## THIMEROSAL IN VACCINES

### (As of February 2011)

- Tripedia (DTaP, by Sanofi Pasteur)[X]

- Tetanus Toxoid Adsorbed (TT, by Sanofi Pasteur), 0.01 percent[#]

- AFLURIA (multidose flu vaccine, by CSL Ltd), 0.01 percent[#]

- FluLaval (flu vaccine, GlaxoSmithKline), 0.01 percent[#]

- Fluvirin (multidose flu vaccine, Novartis), 0.01 percent[#]

- Fluvirin (prefilled syringe, flu vaccine, Novartis)[X]

- Fluzone (5 mL vial, Sanofi Pasteur), 0.01 percent[#]

- JE-VAX (Japanese encephalitis, Sanofi Pasteur), 0.007 percent

- Menomune (multi-dose, meningococcal, Sanofi Pasteur), 0.01 percent[#]

- Pediarix (DTaP-HepB-IPV, GlaxoSmithKline), less than 12.5 nanograms of mercury

x Although this product is considered to be thimerosal-free, the vaccine may contain trace amounts (less than 0.3 micrograms) of mercury remaining after post-production removal of thimerosal. This amount reportedly has no biological effect, but some people dispute this claim.

\# A concentration of 1:10,000 is equivalent to a 0.01 percent concentration. Thimerosal is approximately 50 percent mercury by weight. A 1:10,000 concentration contains 25 micrograms of mercury per 0.5 mL, which is the standard pediatric dose. In the case of AFLURIA, the amount of mercury is 24.5 micrograms of mercury per 0.5 mL.

## Aluminum

Aluminum is the most commonly licensed adjuvant added to children's vaccines. Although the pharmaceutical industry and various government agencies, including the Food and Drug Administration, insist aluminum is safe to add to vaccines, not everyone agrees.

Pediatrician Lawrence B. Palevsky, MD, FAAP, is among those who do not. In an article he wrote titled "Aluminum and Vaccine Ingredients: What Do We Know? What Don't We Know?" he pointed out that as far back as 1996 the American Academy of Pediatrics issued a position paper on aluminum toxicity in infants and children and in the very first paragraph it stated: "Aluminum is now being implicated as interfering with a variety of cellular and metabolic processes in the nervous system and in other tissues."

Dr. Palevsky notes there is "a surprising lack of scientific evidence that injected aluminum is safe" and a "limited understanding of what happens to children when aluminum is injected into their bodies." Even more disconcerting to Dr. Palevsky is the "lack of accepted scientific data explaining whether injected aluminum interacts with other vaccine ingredients to cause harm to our children."

He notes the work of Boyd Haley, PhD, professor emeritus of chemistry at the University of Kentucky, who conducted lab experiments that showed how nerve cells are damaged when they are exposed to aluminum, especially when other ingredients found in vaccines, such as mercury, formaldehyde, and neomycin, are also present. Dr. Haley presented his concerns to the House of Representatives and the Honorable Dan Burton, chairman of the Committee on Government Reform, in May 2001.

However, notes Dr. Palevsky, Haley's data has not been heeded by government institutions that make vaccine policies. Palevsky warns that aluminum is added to vaccines so they will cause a more potent antibody response and that "it is this role as an adjuvant that may reveal to us the most significant relationship between aluminum in vaccines and the damage it imparts on the long term health of our children's nervous and immune systems."

More recently, there has been concern expressed about the use of aluminum in vaccines given to military personnel required to be vaccinated against anthrax. In the 2009 article, the investigators injected mice with adjuvants, including aluminum hydroxide, that were the same as those in the anthrax vaccine. The mice showed both behavioral and motor deficits, a decline in the number of motor neurons, and an increase in the death of neurons. When another group of mice was given a series of aluminum hydroxide injections over two weeks, the investigators reported that the injections caused "profound effects on motor and other behaviors," including memory problems. The investigators concluded that "overall, the results reported here mirror previous work that has clearly demonstrated that aluminum, in both oral and injected forms, can be neurotoxic."

## DO DOCTORS GIVE TOO MANY VACCINES AND TOO SOON?

New parents typically have a long list of questions and concerns regarding their newest addition to the family, and among them are those about vaccines. *Is it safe for my infant to be getting vaccines right after birth and during the first few months to a year of life? At what age does a child's immune system reach maturity? More specifically, when does a child's immune system mature enough to handle vaccinations, whether it's one or several at a time?* These seemingly simple questions have no simple answers and, in fact, elicit a variety of answers from different experts. Here are some thoughts on the matter for you to ponder.

## Paul A. Offit, MD

According to a study conducted by Paul A. Offit, MD, chief of Infectious Diseases and director of the Vaccine Education Center at The Children's Hospital of Philadelphia, and his colleagues, an infant's immune system is capable of handling vaccines immediately after birth. In the 2002 study, Offit reported: "The infant immune system has an enormous capacity to respond safely and effectively to immune system challenges from vaccines."

In a report titled "Addressing Parents' Concerns: Do Multiple Vaccines Overwhelm or Weaken the Infant Immune System?" Dr. Offit says that newborns are able to generate a protective immune response to bacteria, viruses, and vaccines from the time they are born. He claims that "our analysis shows that infants have the theoretical capacity to respond to about 10,000 vaccines at once. Currently, the most vaccines that children receive at one time is five."

Although infants and young children today are given more vaccines than were children decades ago, they actually receive fewer substances in vaccines that stimulate an immune response than they once did, explains Dr. Offit. "Whereas previously one vaccine, smallpox, contained about 200 antigens, now the 11 routinely recommended childhood vaccines contain fewer than 130 antigens combined."

Dr. Offit also dismisses the belief that infants or children who have a mild or moderate illness are more likely to have an adverse reaction to a vaccine than are healthy children. "Studies have found that the presence of a minor to moderate illness such as an upper respiratory tract infection, ear infection, skin infection, fever or diarrhea does not compromise a child's ability to respond to vaccine or increase the risk of an adverse vaccine reaction."

## Lawrence B. Palevsky, MD, FAAP

Lawrence B. Palevsky, MD, a Fellow of the American Academy of Pediatrics (FAAP), cofounder and president of the Holistic Pediatric Association, and past president of the American Holistic Medical Association, sees a child's immune system as maturing later. He offered his views on the immune system, vaccinations, and their ingredients in a piece titled "Aluminum and Vaccine Ingredients: What Do We Know? What Don't We Know?"

In it he explained that children are born with what is called a cellular mediated immune system, a humoral immune system, and a regulator immune system, all of which are major components of their overall immune systems. Each of these major components is composed of specialized cells, referred to as TH cells: TH1, TH2, and TH3. When infants are born, the three parts of the immune system are immature, but they begin to mature as babies are exposed to and interact with their environment.

According to Palevsky, "Antibiotics, poor nutrition, stress, exposure to heavy metals and other environmental toxins, and the use of vaccines, may interfere with the proper maturing process of these three arms of children's immune systems. In theory, if the TH system is allowed to mature, and is not interfered with, children will develop a mature, balanced TH1, TH2 and TH3 immune system by age three."

Parents who are concerned about their children being vaccinated at too young an age can weigh the research, discuss their concerns with knowledgeable professionals, and consider alternative vaccination scheduling, which I discuss in the chapter 15 "Action Plan."

## Stephanie Cave, MS, MD, FAAFP

Pediatrician Stephanie Cave has been a longtime advocate of safe vaccines for children and has treated thousands of children with autism in her practice. In her book, *What Your Doctor May Not Tell You About Children's Vaccinations,* on the issue of the immune system and vaccines, she notes: "Some experts claim that the immune system responds to live, attenuated vaccines the same way it does to a natural infection; others disagree. In fact, even proponents of live vaccines agree that live vaccines can cause a mild version of the disease they are designed to prevent. People who question the wisdom of giving live vaccines, especially to infants and young children, say these vaccines may have much more serious consequences, pointing to the correlation with autism and autoimmune diseases." Dr. Cave is a proponent of alternative vaccination schedules as a way to address parents' concerns about vaccine safety. (See chapter 15, "Action Plan.")

## DOES THE MMR VACCINE INCREASE THE RISK OF AUTISM?

Perhaps the most well-known controversy surrounding the MMR vaccine is its reported link with autism. In 1998, the medical journal *Lancet* published the findings of Andrew Wakefield, MBBS, and his colleagues, who suggested a link existed between the MMR vaccine and autism. Briefly, Wakefield and his colleagues studied twelve children who they said had gastrointestinal problems and developmental regression that began one to fourteen days after they received the MMR vaccine. The researchers suggested the vaccine caused the gastrointestinal syndrome in susceptible children and that the syndrome triggered autism.

Following an investigation by the UK General Medical Council and investigative reporter Brian Deer, Wakefield's study was ruled to be a fraud and he and his senior research advisor were stripped of their medical licenses. Some of the main problems with the study, as noted in the *British Medical Journal,* included the following:

- The children in the study were recruited through an anti-MMR-vaccine campaign.

- Wakefield did not disclose that he was being paid by a UK attorney who was suing MMR vaccine makers for damages.

- Despite being described as "previously normal," five of the children in the study had evidence of developmental issues before they were given the MMR vaccine.

- For all twelve children, their parents' accounts and medical records contradict case descriptions in Wakefield's published study.

- Only one of the twelve children in the study had regressive autism, even though the study stated that nine had the condition. Three of these nine children were never diagnosed with autism.

In a statement published in the February 6, 2010, issue of *The Lancet,* the editors said: "Following the judgment of the UK General Medical Council's Fitness to Practice Panel on Jan 28, 2010, it has become clear that several elements of the 1998 paper by Wakefield et al. are incorrect, contrary to the findings of an earlier investigation. In particular, the claims in the original paper that children were 'consecutively referred' and that investigations were 'approved' by the local ethics committee have been proven to be false. Therefore we fully retract this paper from the published record."

In addition, a comprehensive inquiry by UK investigative reporter Brian Deer found that Wakefield deliberately faked the study's findings and an editorial in the *British Medical*

*Journal* noted: "Deer unearthed evidence of clear falsifica-
tion. Who perpetrated this fraud? There is no doubt that it
was Wakefield's."

Despite these reports of fraud, some parents continue to
believe that the MMR vaccine may cause autism. As proof,
some refer to cases in which the U.S. government has offered compensation to parents whose children have suffered
developmental delays ruled to be associated with vaccinations. In addition, some researchers offer evidence that the
case is far from closed. For more on a possible link between
MMR and autism (beyond the Wakefield connection), see
"MMR and Autism: Another Possibility," in chapter 9.

## HERD IMMUNITY: HOW SAFE IS IT?

I introduced the concept of herd immunity in chapter 1 when
discussing the infant's immune system, but relying on herd
immunity can also be an ethical issue. For sure, one way to
protect your infant from infectious diseases is to make sure
the people who are close to your child have been immunized.
Besides the hepatitis B vaccine, which is recommended for
newborns, infants do not begin to receive their other recommended vaccine series until they are at least 6 to 8 weeks old.
Even then, one dose of a vaccine is not sufficient for an infant
to build up resistance.

Therefore, the best thing you can do is know who has
been properly vaccinated—other children in the family,
grandparents, uncle and aunts, cousins, other family members, and friends—if they are going to be around your infant. Individuals who are protected against the diseases will
not pass them along to your infant. As a parent, you can ask
your family and friends to help you exercise this caution.

Herd immunity can be more of an ethical issue, however,
when parents rely on it when sending an unvaccinated child
to school. Lack of complete vaccination coverage for a specific disease increases the risk of the disease for the whole
population, including the people who have been vaccinated,

because it reduces herd immunity. However, complete vaccination coverage does not exist except in selected groups; say, all the children in one third-grade class in your child's school may be fully immunized even if your child is not. Yet your child could then go to a large family gathering where one or more people have not been vaccinated. In that situation, herd immunity would offer less protection than in the classroom situation.

If you have a child who has not achieved immunity against any of the childhood diseases, for whatever reason, you need to consider what impact herd immunity may have on your child's health. It can be helpful to discuss your concerns with a trusted medical professional. (See "Finding the Right Physician" in chapter 15.)

## HOW DO PARENTS FEEL ABOUT VACCINE SAFETY?

Finally, I thought I would end this chapter with a look at how parents feel about vaccine safety. In June 2011, the results of a survey, which were analyzed by researchers at the Centers for Disease Control and Prevention and the Department of Health and Human Services National Vaccine Program Office, found that while most children in the United States are getting their regularly scheduled immunizations, a number of parents believe some or all vaccines are not safe or necessary.

The investigators questioned 376 households about vaccines. Only 23 percent of parents said they had no worries about vaccines, while the remaining 77 percent had at least one question or concern about their children experiencing physical pain from shots, getting too many shots in one visit, getting too many vaccines before 2 years of age, and receiving vaccines that contain unsafe ingredients. Parents also wondered if vaccines were being tested enough or if they might cause chronic disease.

About 2 percent of parents said they would not allow their children to get any of the recommended vaccines, and

5 percent said they would choose some but not all vaccines for their children.

Several things are important about these survey results. One, if you have concerns about vaccinations, you have plenty of company, and so there are many others with whom you can share information and your concerns. Two, these findings raise awareness that while the vast majority of parents accept that vaccinations are critical, they are also aware vaccines are not as safe as they could or should be. As more and more parents raise their voices about vaccine safety to vaccine makers and policy makers, it is hoped vaccines will become a safer, more effective way to fight childhood diseases.

# CHAPTER 3

Hepatitis B

Shortly after most children in the United States enter the world, they are greeted with the first of a long series of vaccinations. At the head of that list is the vaccine for hepatitis B, which is a vaccine that has met with considerable success but has also stirred up its share of controversy.

According to the Hepatitis B Foundation, the virus is one hundred times more infectious than the AIDS virus, yet, unlike AIDS, there is an effective vaccine that can prevent hepatitis B. For the more than 1 million Americans who are chronically infected with hepatitis B, the vaccine is of no help. But for the nearly one hundred thousand people who become newly infected each year, the vaccine could make a difference. A significant concern is infants and young children: while most healthy adults (about 90 percent) who become infected with the virus can recover and develop immunity against future infections, most infants and up to half of young children who become infected go on to develop chronic infections. That is why the vaccines are targeted for the youngest of our population.

So I begin the journey through the world of childhood vaccinations with a close look at the disease the vaccine was designed to prevent.

## WHAT IS HEPATITIS B?

"Hepatitis" is a broad term that means "inflammation of the liver," and it also refers to a family of viral infections that can have a negative impact on liver function. The most common of these infections are hepatitis A, B, and C. For now I am concerned with hepatitis B, which is a contagious liver disease caused by the hepatitis B virus (HBV).

Hepatitis B is a worldwide problem. According to the Hepatitis B Foundation, 2 billion people or one-third of the world's population is infected with hepatitis B. That does not mean every one of these individuals is very ill or even has symptoms, but 400 million are chronically infected.

In the United States, it is estimated that 5 percent (12 million Americans) are infected with the virus, and about five thousand people die from hepatitis B and its complications every year. The good news is that the rate of acute hepatitis B in the United States has declined a dramatic 82 percent since 1990, which was when vaccination of children for hepatitis B was initiated.

### Types of Hepatitis B

Hepatitis B can appear in two forms: acute and chronic. Symptoms of acute hepatitis B usually appear an average of ninety days after someone has been exposed to HBV, but this can range from six weeks to six months. Most individuals who get acute hepatitis B experience symptoms for only a few weeks, but the symptoms can linger for as long as six months for some people. Ninety to 95 percent of adults who develop acute hepatitis B fight off the disease. About 5 to 10 percent develop chronic hepatitis B, an infection with HBV that lasts longer than six months and often is a lifelong condition associated with serious health problems, even death.

Children, however, have a much greater risk for developing chronic hepatitis B; in fact, up to 90 percent of infants who become infected with HBV cannot eliminate the virus and end up with chronic hepatitis B.

## Symptoms of Hepatitis B

It is difficult to know exactly how many people have hepatitis B because about 30 to 50 percent of people with the virus, including children, do not experience symptoms and so do not seek medical help. However, among those who do have symptoms, they can include the following:

- Dark urine

- Loss of appetite

- Jaundice (yellowing of the eyes and/or skin)

- Fatigue

- Nausea and vomiting

- Itching all over the body

- Gray or pale-colored stools

- Pain on the right side of the abdomen, under the lower rib cage

If you have hepatitis B without symptoms, you can still spread the virus to other people. Most people who have hepatitis B remain symptom-free for decades. About 15 to 25 percent of people who have chronic hepatitis B eventually develop serious problems such as liver cancer or cirrhosis. Even then, however, they may not display symptoms until the disease is at its late stages, although blood tests for liver function can reveal abnormalities in the liver and alert you to problems with the liver.

## How Hepatitis B Is Transmitted

Hepatitis B is transmitted from an infected person to someone who is free of the virus through bodily fluids, such as semen or blood. The disease is more often spread through sexual contact, which accounts for about two-thirds of all cases of hepatitis. Hepatitis B is also transmitted by sharing needles or other drug injection paraphernalia. One more way of transmitting the disease is from an infected mother to her infant during childbirth. This form of transmission, however, is not common. (See "Hepatitis B and Pregnancy.")

It's also important to note the ways hepatitis B is **not** transmitted. You cannot get hepatitis B by sharing eating utensils, hugging, kissing, coughing, sneezing, holding hands, or breast-feeding or from toilet seats.

## Hepatitis B and Pregnancy

If you plan to get pregnant or are pregnant, you should be tested for hepatitis B. Testing is a simple matter: a quick blood test will show if you have a special protein called an antigen that indicates you have the virus. If you do have HBV,

### HEPATITIS FACT

Hepatitis A, B, and C are caused by three different viruses. Although each virus can cause similar symptoms, they also have different effects on the liver. Hepatitis A does not become chronic and usually goes away without treatment. Both hepatitis B and C can begin as short-term infections (acute) but result in chronic disease and long-term liver problems. There are vaccines to prevent hepatitis A and B but not hepatitis C.

your health-care provider will do additional tests to determine if your liver is healthy. You should also inform anyone in your household and your sexual partner(s) that you have the virus, because they are at risk of contracting hepatitis B and should be tested.

If you contract the disease while pregnant, there is a chance you will infect your child. According to the American College of Obstetricians and Gynecologists, about 1 in every 500 to 1,000 pregnant women has hepatitis when she gives birth.[2] The risk of an infant contracting hepatitis from his or her mother is less than 10 percent if the woman develops the disease early in pregnancy and up to 90 percent if she gets the disease late in pregnancy.

## Risk Factors for Hepatitis B

Risk factors for hepatitis B include the following:

- Having more than one sex partner in six months

- Using intravenous drugs

- Receiving blood transfusions or being on dialysis

- Working in public safety or health care where you are exposed to infected bodily fluids

- Being in the military or traveling to high-risk areas

- Living with someone who has chronic hepatitis B

## Hepatitis B in Infants

Infants who contract hepatitis B from their mothers are at risk for severe health problems. Up to 90 percent of newborns infected with hepatitis B from their mothers will develop chronic disease, and they have a 25 percent risk of dying of liver cancer or cirrhosis of the liver when they reach adulthood. Infected babies can also transmit the virus to other people.

## ABOUT THE HEPATITIS B VACCINES

In 1991, the U.S. government issued guidelines recommending three doses of the hepatitis B vaccine for every child born after 1990, as well as for certain adult populations, which I discuss later. The hepatitis B vaccine is an intramuscular injection that is usually administered as a series of three doses. The vaccines are available as a single product under the names Engerix-B (made by GlaxoSmithKline) and Recombivax HB (made by Merck).

Both vaccines are prepared synthetically and do not contain blood products; therefore, it is not possible to get hepatitis B from these vaccines. Also, for those concerned about thimerosal, the preservative that is 49.6 percent mercury (read about thimerosal in chapter 16), all of the pediatric formulations of hepatitis B vaccines were licensed to be thimerosal-free (Recombivax HB in August 1999 and Engerix-B in January 2007).

**Question: Is it safe for my child to get two different brands of the hepatitis B vaccine during the three-dose series?**

A controlled study showed that completing the course of immunization with one dose of Engerix-B month 6 after children received doses one and two of Recombivax HB was safe and provided the same degree of protection against hepatitis B as did receiving three doses of Recombivax HB at months 0, 1, and 6. You and your doctor should discuss any possibilities that your child may need to switch to another brand of hepatitis B vaccine.

Hepatitis B is also available in combination vaccines that include other common childhood vaccinations; for example, COMVAX (contains Hib and Hep B) and PEDIARIX (contains DTaP+Hep B+IPV [polio]). The COMVAX vaccine is discussed in chapter 6, and details about PEDIARIX are in chapter 5.

## Engerix-B

The Engerix-B vaccine is a noninfectious vaccine made from hepatitis B surface antigen (HBsAg) obtained by culturing genetically engineered yeast cells called *Saccharomyces cerevisiae,* which carry the surface antigen gene of the hepatitis B virus. In addition to the HBsAg antigen, each pediatric and adolescent dose contains 0.25 milligrams of aluminum hydroxide, sodium chloride and phosphate buffers (disodium phosphate dehydrate, sodium dihydrogen phosphate dehydrate), and no more than 5 percent yeast protein. The vaccine is provided in prefilled syringes with a tip cap and/or rubber plunger that may contain natural latex rubber. These syringes can cause allergic reactions in infants and children who are sensitive to latex.

## Recombivax HB

The Recombivax HB hepatitis B vaccine is a noninfectious vaccine derived from hepatitis B surface antigen (HBsAg) produced from cultures of a recombinant yeast strain, *Saccharomyces cerevisiae.* In addition to the antigen, each 0.5 mL dose contains approximately 0.5 mg of aluminum hydroxyphosphate sulfate and may contain no more than 1 percent yeast protein. The vaccine also contains less than 15 mcg/mL residual formaldehyde, but it does not contain preservatives.

Recombivax HB is provided for intramuscular injection. However, it can be given subcutaneously if your child is at risk of hemorrhage.

## Who Should Get the Hepatitis B Vaccine?

The Centers for Disease Control and Prevention and the American Academy of Pediatrics recommend that all infants and children be vaccinated against hepatitis B. In addition, the CDC recommends that adults who are in high-risk groups be vaccinated.

You may notice that the list of people who should be vaccinated against hepatitis B corresponds closely with the list of risk factors for the disease. That's because hepatitis B is transmitted between people and so the types of interactions you and your children have with certain groups of people have a significant impact on who should be vaccinated. Therefore, here is a general guide for vaccination:

- All newborns at birth and all children up to age 18 years

- Sexually active teens and adults

- Health-care professionals and medical emergency personnel

- Sex partners and/or close family/household members who live with an infected individual

- Anyone who has kidney disease or who is undergoing dialysis

- Residents and staff of group homes and correctional institutions

- Anyone who travels to countries where hepatitis B is common (e.g., Asia, Africa, Eastern Europe, Middle East, Pacific islands, South America)

- People who are considering adoption, domestic or international

Forty-seven states and the District of Columbia require vaccination for hepatitis B before children can enter school. The three states that do not have this requirement are Alabama, Montana, and South Dakota. See the Immunization Action Coalition entry in the appendices for links to specific information for each state.

## The Hepatitis B Schedule

The CDC 2010 vaccination schedule for children is as follows:

- The initial shot is given to infants before they leave the hospital. If the mother is a carrier of hepatitis B, the infant should be given the first dose of the vaccine shortly after birth, along with an injection of hepatitis B immune globulin (see "Hepatitis B Immune Globulin"). The first dose of hepatitis B vaccine may be given at the same time as the immune globulin, but it should be administered in the opposite thigh.

- The second shot is administered one month after the first dose.

- The third shot is given at least two months after the second dose and at least four months after the first dose.

You can discuss alternative vaccination dosing with your physician. If an infant does not receive the first shot until age 4 to 8 weeks, for example, the second shot is administered at 4 months and the third at 6 to 16 months. Even when hepatitis B vaccines are given according to this alternative schedule, the other routine childhood immunizations should still be followed. Yet another option is a four-dose schedule that has been approved for Engerix-B for administration at 0, 1, 2, and 12 months of age.

Adolescents who have never received the hepatitis B

vaccine series should be vaccinated as soon as possible. Adolescents ages 11 through 15 years may follow the two-dose schedule of Recombivax HB, which has been approved for this age group. According to this schedule, after the first dose of Recombivax HB is given the second dose is administered four to six months later.

## Hepatitis B Immune Globulin

Infants who are born to mothers infected with HBV are also given hepatitis B immune globulin (e.g., BayHep B, Nabi-HB). Hepatitis B immune globulin is made from human plasma (a blood product) and contains proteins that protect the infant against inflammation of the liver. Although all donated human plasma is tested and treated to reduce the risk of transmitting disease, the possibility still exists, so you should discuss the risks and benefits of giving your infant hepatitis B immune globulin with your physician.

Even though hepatitis B immune globulin is not a vaccine, it does help prevent transmission of hepatitis B in 80 to 90 percent of cases when it is given along with the hepatitis B vaccine. The recommended time to administer hepatitis B immune globulin is within twelve hours of birth or when the infant is medically stable. It is given as an injection into a muscle or intravenously.

Infants born to mothers who have hepatitis B are not the only young people who may need hepatitis B immune globulin. Other children and adolescents who have somehow been exposed to HBV through blood (e.g., transfusion, needles) or because someone close to them has acute hepatitis B may need to receive immune globulin as well.

## Side Effects of Hepatitis B Immune Globulin

Aside from the hepatitis B vaccine, hepatitis B immune globulin is associated with its own side effects. Those that require immediate medical attention are not common but can include an allergic reaction (e.g., hives, breathing difficulties, swelling of the face, lips, tongue, or throat), increased blood pressure (characterized by severe headache, blurry vision, chest pain, numbness, seizures), nausea, low fever, loss of appetite, dark urine, clay-colored stools, and jaundice. Less serious side effects may include diarrhea, tremors or shaking, back or joint pain, upset stomach, chills, and tiredness.

## When to Delay or Avoid the Hepatitis B Vaccine

For infants and children who are ill with an ailment that is more serious than a cold getting the vaccine should be delayed until they have recovered. Any child who has a severe allergic reaction to baker's yeast should not get the vaccine, and no child who has responded to the vaccine with a serious allergic reaction should get any further injections of hepatitis B vaccine.

You should also consult your physician before your child is administered the hepatitis B vaccine if he or she has any of the following conditions:

- Kidney disease

- Multiple sclerosis

- A bleeding or blood-clotting disorder such as hemophilia

- An allergy to latex rubber

- A history of seizures

- A neurological condition that affects the brain

- An immune system compromised by a bone marrow transplant or disease

Before your child is given the hepatitis B vaccine, tell your doctor if he or she has received drugs or treatments within the past two weeks that may weaken the immune system. Your child may not be able to receive the vaccine or may need to wait until the other treatments are finished before getting immunized. The drugs may include:

- Any form of steroid medications

- Blood thinners

- Chemotherapy

- Medications to treat autoimmune disorders, such as azathioprine, efalizumab, etanercept, leflunomide, and others

- Medications to treat or prevent organ transplant rejection, such as basiliximab, cyclosporine, muromonab-CD3, mycophenolate mofetil, sirolimus, or tacrolimus

- There may be other drugs that can affect the hepatitis B vaccine, so make sure to tell your doctor about any over-the-counter or prescription medications, as well as natural supplements, your child may be taking.

## Side Effects of the Hepatitis B Vaccine

Most infants who receive the hepatitis B vaccine do not experience side effects. The CDC reports that about 25 percent of recipients experience soreness at the injection site and a fever of 99.9°F or greater occurs in about 1 in 15 people. Other less serious side effects may include:

- Pain and/or redness at the injection site

- Dizziness, headache

- Joint pain

- Body aches

- Gastrointestinal disorders, such as constipation, diarrhea, nausea, stomach pain, vomiting

- Tiredness

Serious adverse reactions are rare and usually associated with an allergic reaction to a component of the vaccine. The CDC states that such responses occur in 1 in 1.1 million doses. If any of the following serious side effects occur, you should contact your health-care provider immediately:

- Fussiness, irritability, and/or crying for an hour or longer

- Fever, sore throat, and headache accompanied by a blistering red skin rash that peels

- Fast or pounding heartbeat

- Easy bruising or bleeding

For additional information about side effects and reactions to hepatitis B vaccine, see "Concerns and Controversies."

According to GlaxoSmithKline, the makers of Engerix-B, apnea (pauses in breathing) following intramuscular vaccination has been seen in some premature infants. If your child was born prematurely, the decision to give him or her an intramuscular vaccine such as Engerix-B should be made after you discuss the potential risks and benefits of vaccination with your health-care provider.

## CONCERNS AND CONTROVERSIES

The controversies about administering hepatitis B vaccine
to newborns and children revolve mainly around two issues:
whether it is necessary to immunize newborns and young
children against a disease to which they are rarely exposed
and whether the vaccine is safe; that is, does immunization
place children at increased risk of developing certain diseases, such as multiple sclerosis and other neurological disorders, as some have claimed? Let's look at each of these
two concerns separately.

### Is the Hepatitis B Vaccine Necessary?

One of the concerns raised by some parents and medical
professionals regarding the hepatitis B vaccine is that because hepatitis B is rarely seen in children and is largely a
disease associated with sexual activity and/or illicit drug
use there is no need to vaccinate newborns or young children against this disease, unless the mother has tested positive for the disease. Prenatal testing for hepatitis B is
generally routine and simple, and so identifying which infants would need immunization could be known ahead of
delivery.

Support for not administering the hepatitis B vaccine to
newborns and young children goes back more than a decade. According to Jane Orient, MD, an internist who made
a statement on behalf of the Association of American Physicians & Surgeons to the Subcommittee on Criminal Justice,
Drug Policy and Human Resources of the Committee on
Government Reform in the U.S. House of Representatives in
1999, "Information given to parents about this vaccine often
does not meet the requirement for full disclosure. For example, it may state 'getting the disease is far more likely to
cause serious illness than getting the vaccine.' This may be
literally true, but it is seriously misleading if the risk of getting the disease is nearly zero (as is true for most American

newborns)." Dr. Orient also noted that "for most children, the risk of a serious vaccine reaction may be 100 times greater than the risk of hepatitis B."

Dr. Bob Sears, author of *The Vaccine Book: Making the Right Decision for Your Child,* recommends not giving the hepatitis B vaccine to newborns immediately after birth. Instead, he suggests delaying the first shot for the first two months because (1) the shot can cause fever, lethargy, and poor feeding; and (2) the disease is sexually transmitted and so does not occur in newborns.

Some parents are reacting against the recommendation to vaccinate their infants with HBV. At an October 2010 meeting of the Infectious Diseases Society of America, for example, researchers presented their findings from a study that used data gathered from hospitals in Colorado for the year 2008. A total of 39,703 infants in the study (61.6 percent) had received a dose of HBV at birth. The researchers found that white mothers were significantly more likely to refuse the HBV vaccine than Hispanics and that the same held true for mothers with a master's degree versus those with an eighth-grade education. The findings of this study have led some people to comment that better-educated mothers are more likely to refuse the vaccine for their infants because they are more informed about the risks.

## Is the Hepatitis B Vaccine Safe?

The safety of hepatitis B vaccine has been evaluated by the Centers for Disease Control and Prevention, the World Health Organization, and various professional medical associations. They report there is no evidence that the vaccine causes multiple sclerosis, sudden infant death syndrome (SIDS), or other neurological disorders. Not everyone agrees.

One of the health conditions that has been associated with hepatitis B vaccine is multiple sclerosis. For example:

- A study conducted by experts from the Harvard School of Public Health using a database from the

United Kingdom evaluated a potential link between the hepatitis B vaccine and an increased risk of multiple sclerosis between January 1993 and December 2000. A total of 163 individuals with multiple sclerosis and 1,604 controls were studied, and the investigators found a 3.1% increased risk of developing multiple sclerosis within three years of receiving the vaccine. They did not, however, see an increased risk of multiple sclerosis associated with getting either the tetanus or influenza vaccinations. The authors of this study were not able to determine if the vaccine triggered the disease in people who were already susceptible or if it caused the disease to present itself sooner.

- A subsequent study published in *Neurology* in 2009 reported an increased risk of developing central nervous system inflammatory demyelination—a characteristic of multiple sclerosis—among children who received the hepatitis B vaccine compared with children who did not. The trend was especially high (2.77 times the risk) among patients with confirmed multiple sclerosis and who received the Engerix B vaccine. The authors noted in their conclusions that while hepatitis B vaccination does not usually increase the risk of central nervous system inflammatory demyelination in children, the Engerix B vaccine appeared to do so, and they encouraged additional studies.

In addition to multiple sclerosis, some medical professionals have suggested that type 1 diabetes may be linked to the hepatitis B vaccine. For example:

- In a New Zealand study, investigators reported the incidence of type 1 diabetes rose 60 percent among children after there was a mass hepatitis B immunization campaign in the country.

- In 2000 at the annual meeting of the American Diabetes Association, a group of scientists reported that children who receive hepatitis B vaccine are at greater risk for developing type 1 diabetes than those who are never vaccinated. In Italy, Paolo Pozzilli, MD, and his colleagues compared 150,000 children who had been vaccinated at age 3 months with an equal number of unvaccinated children. They also looked at 400,000 children who received the vaccination at age 12 when vaccination became mandatory in Italy and compared them with children who had not been vaccinated. Among the children who were vaccinated at age 3 months the rate of type 1 diabetes was 46 per 100,000 children, and among those not vaccinated it was 34 per 100,000. In the older children, the rates were 17.8 per 100,000 for vaccinated children and 6.9 per 100,000 for unvaccinated children.

Hepatitis B vaccine has also been named as a possible player in autism. Researchers from the State University of New York at Stony Brook conducted a study using data from the National Health Interview Survey 1997–2002 and evaluated the odds of developing autism associated with neonatal hepatitis B vaccination among boys ages 3 to 17 years. Analysis of the data showed that boys vaccinated as neonates had a threefold greater risk of getting a diagnosis of autism than boys who were never vaccinated or who were vaccinated after age 1 month. Non-Hispanic white boys were 64 percent less likely to develop autism than nonwhite boys. The authors published their findings in the *Journal of Toxicology and Environmental Health*.

## Hepatitis B Vaccine Reactions in Adults

Although my discussion is primarily about children, it is worth noting some research on possible reactions to the hepatitis B vaccine in adults, as the findings may have relevance to the young. In a study published in the *Annals of Pharmacotherapy,* investigators report on the incidence of reactions to hepatitis B vaccine administered to an estimated 20,516,508 adults, according to data from the Centers for Disease Control and Prevention, from 1997 through 2000. As a control group, the researchers used data concerning 141,832,679 adults who received a tetanus-diphtheria injection from 1991 through 2000.

The investigators found that adults who were vaccinated against hepatitis B were at risk for developing acute cases of arthritis, gastrointestinal disease, multiple sclerosis, myelitis, neuritis, neuropathy, and thrombocytopenia and that some patients went on to experience adverse reactions for a year or longer. In subsequent studies, the findings were similar: adults who received hepatitis B vaccine showed a significantly increased risk for multiple sclerosis, optic neurotis, vasculitis, arthritis, alopecia (hair loss), lupus erythematosus, rheumatoid arthritis, and thrombocytopenia.

# CHAPTER 4

Rotavirus

In June 2009, the World Health Organization recommended that a vaccine designed to prevent diarrhea and dehydration associated with rotavirus be part of national immunization programs around the world. In June 2011, two large vaccine makers, GlaxoSmithKline and Merck, announced they were reducing the prices they charged developing countries for the rotavirus vaccine by 68 percent. These two moves were critically important, because each year more than five hundred thousand children die from diarrheal diseases caused by rotavirus and an additional 2 million require hospitalization. Although most of the deaths associated with rotavirus occur in developing countries, children anywhere in the world can be exposed to and develop life-threatening rotavirus-related diarrhea and dehydration, especially infants and children younger than 2 years old.

Before 2006, rotavirus was the main cause of severe diarrhea among infants and young children in the United States. That's the year the rotavirus vaccine was introduced in the States. During the years before the vaccine was recommended to be administered to all infants, some significant figures were associated with rotavirus: more than 400,000 doctor visits, more than 200,000 emergency department visits, up to 70,000 hospitalizations, and 20 to 60 deaths in children younger than 5 years of age occurred each year.

Let's look at what rotavirus is and how it can be prevented.

## WHAT IS ROTAVIRUS?

Rotavirus is one of the most common causes of diarrhea, and a severe form of the disease, called rotavirus gastroenteritis, is the main cause of severe, dehydrating diarrhea in infants and young children. Each year in the United States, about 3 million cases of diarrhea develop in children younger than 5 years old and approximately fifty-five thousand require hospitalization for the diarrhea and dehydration. The good news about rotavirus infection in the United States is that very few deaths are related to the disease. For that positive note we can largely thank the rotavirus vaccine.

### Symptoms of Rotavirus

Rotavirus causes inflammation of the intestinal tract and stomach (a condition known as gastroenteritis). The first indication that an infant or young child has rotavirus is a fever, which is followed by three to eight days of watery diarrhea and vomiting. Abdominal pain may develop as well. If your child develops severe or bloody diarrhea, experiences vomiting that lasts for more than three hours, has a fever that reaches 103°F or higher, seems lethargic or in pain, and/or has indications that he or she is dehydrated—dry mouth, crying without tears, little or no urine output, and/or unusual tiredness or unresponsiveness—take your child to a doctor as soon as possible. Although most cases of rotavirus infection are mild, about 2 percent of children develop severe dehydration.

### How Rotavirus Is Transmitted

Rotavirus is highly contagious. The rotavirus is shed in feces of infected individuals and spread when the virus enters the mouth of another person. This way of transmitting the virus is called the fecal-oral route. Because rotavirus can survive for days on dry and hard surfaces and can live for hours on human hands, it is important that children and anyone who has contact with children wash their hands often.

Even a minute amount of fecal matter on the hands can transmit the virus to other children (or to adults) or to toys and other objects children put in their mouth. Children and adults who touch a contaminated surface can transmit the virus to their mouth. Therefore it is essential that children wash their hands after using the toilet and before eating. Anyone who changes diapers or who helps young children with toileting should also wash their hands. Rotavirus can enter the body in food and water, and it also can be transmitted both before and after a child becomes ill with diarrhea.

## Risk Factors for Rotavirus

Children most likely to become infected with rotavirus are those between the ages of 4 and 24 months, especially if they spend time in child-care environments. Others who are at increased risk for rotavirus are older adults and adults who care for young children. The risk for rotavirus infection for all susceptible people in the United States is greatest in the fall months in the Southwest and spreads to the Northeast by the spring months, which means infections are most common from November to May. However, rotavirus infections can occur at any time during the year.

## Treatment of Rotavirus

Because antibiotics are not effective against viruses, treatment of rotavirus typically involves drinking enough fluids (avoid fruit juice and soda) to prevent dehydration and getting enough nourishment if the child is vomiting. Infants or toddlers who become moderately or severely dehydrated may need to get intravenous fluids at a hospital. Some doctors prescribe special drinks to help children replace lost body fluids and nutrients. Over-the-counter medications to treat nausea and vomiting should be avoided unless recommended by your health-care provider.

## ABOUT THE ROTAVIRUS VACCINES

As of 2011, there were two rotavirus vaccines licensed for use in the United States: RotaTeq (Merck), which was licensed in 2006; and ROTARIX (GlaxoSmithKline), which was licensed in 2008. A previous rotavirus vaccine, RotaShield, was withdrawn from the market in 1999 after it was associated with an increase in the number of children who developed intussusception, a serious bowel disease. That vaccine led to a threefold increase in occurrence of intussusceptions when compared with children who were not vaccinated.

Before they were licensed, both RotaTeq and ROTARIX were tested in thousands of children to ensure there was no increased risk of intussusception. Although both RotaTeq and ROTARIX have been associated with safety issues, they were minor and were resolved. (See "RotaTeq" and "ROTARIX.")

RotaTeq and ROTARIX were designed to prevent development of rotavirus infections. Neither vaccine can treat active rotavirus that is already in the body.

### RotaTeq

RotaTeq is an attenuated (weakened) live virus vaccine that is gently squeezed into the mouth from a small applicator. In clinical trials, RotaTeq was found to prevent 74 percent of all rotavirus gastroenteritis cases, about 98 percent of severe rotavirus gastroenteritis cases, and about 96 percent of hospitalizations associated with rotavirus infection.

RotaTeq is considered a pentavalent vaccine, which means it contains five rotaviruses produced by reassortment. Reassortment is the mixing of genetic materials from a species into new combinations in different individuals. The rotavirus strains in the vaccine were isolated from both human and bovine (cow) hosts. In February 2006, the Food and Drug Administration approved RotaTeq for use in the United States, which was followed by approval from Health Canada in August 2006 for use in Canada.

Ingredients in RotaTeq include five live rotavirus strains (G1, G2, G3, G4, and P1), as well as sucrose, sodium citrate, sodium phosphate monobasic monohydrate, sodium hydroxide, polysorbate 80, and fetal bovine serum.

In March 2010, RotaTeq was found to contain pieces of genetic material—broken segments of DNA—from pig viruses called circovirus 1 (PCV1) and circovirus 2 (PCV2). This occurred at the same time the other rotavirus vaccine, ROTARIX, was suspended because of contamination. (See "ROTARIX.") Unlike ROTARIX, however, the license for RotaTeq was not temporarily suspended.

## ROTARIX

ROTARIX is an attenuated (weakened) live virus derived from the human 89-12 strain of G1P[8]-type rotavirus and is indicated for the prevention of rotavirus gastroenteritis caused by G1 and non-G1 types (G3, G4, and G9). The vaccine is available in the form of a liquid that is gently squeezed into the mouth from a prefilled oral applicator. Currently there are two types of these applicators, both of which may contain natural rubber latex. Therefore, any child who is allergic to latex should not be given this vaccine, as the applicators may cause allergic reactions.

In March 2010, the Food and Drug Administration announced that ROTARIX was contaminated with a virus from pigs called circovirus 1 (PCV1). Although there was no evidence that the pig virus was a safety risk to humans, use of ROTARIX was suspended until May 2010, when the FDA announced that after careful review it had decided that the vaccine was safe to administer.

In addition to the live virus, the ROTARIX vaccine contains the following ingredients:

- Amino acids

- Dextran

- Dulbecco's Modified Eagle Medium (DMEM), which contains sodium chloride, potassium chloride, magnesium sulfate, ferric (III) nitrate, sodium phosphate, sodium pyruvate, D-glucose, concentrated vitamin solution, L-cystine, L-tyrosine, amino acids solution, L-glutamine, calcium chloride, sodium hydrogen carbonate, phenol red

- Sorbitol

- Sucrose

During the manufacturing process, materials derived from pigs are used, therefore, porcine circovirus type 1 (PCV-1) is present in ROTARIX. The diluent contains calcium carbonate (an antacid), sterile water, and xanthan. ROTARIX does not contain preservatives.

In clinical trials, ROTARIX was found to prevent 87.1 percent of all rotavirus gastroenteritis cases, about 84 percent of severe cases, and from 85 to 100 percent of hospitalizations associated with rotavirus infection.

## Who Should Get the Rotavirus Vaccine

The National Network for Immunization Information states that all full-term infants should begin the rotavirus vaccination series between the ages of 6 and 14 weeks.[2] There are some exceptions. (See "When to Delay or Avoid the Rotavirus Vaccine.") Rotavirus vaccine may be given at the same time as other childhood vaccines scheduled for your child. If your child was born prematurely, consult your physician about when immunization should begin. Rotavirus vaccine is not mandated by the states for entry into school.

## The Rotavirus Schedule

The recommended schedule for RotaTeq is:

- The first dose is given between 6 and 12 weeks of age.

- The second dose is given four to ten weeks after the first dose.

- The third dose is given four to ten weeks after the second dose. The third dose must be administered before 32 weeks of age (about 8 months old).

The recommended schedule for ROTARIX is:

- The first dose is usually given when the child is 6 weeks old.

- The second dose is administered at least four weeks after the first dose, but before the child is 24 weeks old.

Whenever possible, your child should complete his or her vaccination series with the same product; that is, three doses of RotaTeq or two doses of ROTARIX, and not any combination of the two. If, however, you do not know which brand of vaccine was administered first, the subsequent dose(s) should not be delayed. It is recommended that your child be given the vaccine that is available and that he or she receives a total of three doses.

Your doctor may recommend a different dosing schedule for your child. The CDC advises against starting the vaccine series in babies who are older than 14 weeks and 6 days old. If your baby has not received the first dose of rotavirus vaccine by that age, consult your doctor about whether you should follow a "catch-up" schedule.

## After Dosing

If your child vomits or spits up within one or two hours after taking the rotavirus vaccine, contact your doctor. Your child may need to take a replacement dose.

Always wash your hands thoroughly after handling the diapers of a child who has been given a rotavirus vaccine, as small amounts of the virus may be present in the child's stool and it could infect others who make contact with the stool.

## When to Delay or Avoid the Rotavirus Vaccine

Some infants should not be given the rotavirus vaccine at all, while parents should delay the dose for others. Babies for whom the vaccine should be delayed or avoided include the following:

- *Infants who have had a severe allergic reaction to a previous dose of rotavirus vaccine or to any component of a rotavirus vaccine.* Let your doctor know if your baby has ever had any severe allergies, including an allergy to latex. ROTARIX is packaged in a latex applicator.

- *Babies who are moderately or severely ill at the time the vaccination is scheduled.* The illness may include moderate or severe diarrhea, vomiting, fever, or other conditions. You should consult your physician or other knowledgeable health-care provider about whether it is safe for your infant to receive the vaccine.

- *Infants whose immune system may be compromised because of cancer, HIV/AIDS or other immune system diseases (e.g., severe combined immuno-deficiency disease [SCID]), treatment with drugs such as long-term steroids, transplantation, or cancer treatment with medication or radiation.* There is no reliable safety information about response to the rotavirus vaccine in infants who are immunocompromised. It is known, however, that children and adults who have congenital immunodeficiency or who received a transplant can experience severe and potentially deadly rotavirus gastroenteritis.

- *Infants who have a congenital stomach disorder, leukemia, or other blood disease or who have had recent stomach surgery or a blood transfusion.* Consult your physician about whether your child should receive the vaccine. If your child has received blood products, the vaccine should be delayed for six weeks unless that delay will make the child ineligible for vaccination because of age.

- *Infants who have had intussusception from any cause.* These children are at greater risk for getting the serious bowel condition again.

- *Babies who have not received their first rotavirus vaccination by age 8 months.* The rotavirus vaccine is not recommended for children who are age 8 months or older because there is insufficient evidence showing that it is effective in this age group. There is also some evidence that after age 8 months children are more likely to experience adverse reactions to the vaccine, such as fever.

## Side Effects of the Rotavirus Vaccine

In tests of the vaccine, some children who received a dose of rotavirus experienced more minor symptoms such as diarrhea, fever, sore throat, coughing, ear infection, vomiting,

and runny nose than did children who received a placebo.
These side effects typically appear within seven days of
the dose. Other reported side effects include hives and
Kawasaki disease, a serious condition that can affect the
heart. Symptoms of Kawasaki disease may include fever,
rash, red eyes and mouth, swollen glands, and swollen
hands and feet. If not treated, Kawasaki disease can be life
threatening.

Kawasaki disease is a very rare side effect of the rotavirus
vaccine. In sixteen clinical trials of ROTARIX, for example,
there were eighteen (0.035 percent) cases of Kawasaki disease in recipients of the vaccine compared with nine (0.021
percent) among study subjects who received a placebo.
Among the recipients of the ROTARIX vaccine, the time
until Kawasaki symptoms appeared ranged from three days
to nineteen months.

Severe allergic reactions associated with the rotavirus
vaccine are rare but possible, as they are with any vaccine.
Signs of a serious allergic reaction can include breathing
difficulties, dizziness, fainting, hives, hoarseness, paleness,
rapid heartbeat, and wheezing. These signs can occur within
a few minutes to a few hours after your child receives the
dose. If any of these symptoms occur, seek immediate medical attention.

If your child has symptoms of diarrhea, vomiting, severe
stomach pain, blood in the stool, or changes in bowel movements, these may be signs of the life-threatening condition
intussusception. Contact your doctor immediately if your
child displays these symptoms, even if it has been several
weeks since he or she received the vaccine dose.

Deaths possibly related to the rotavirus vaccine are also
very rare. Based on information from eight clinical trials
reported by the manufacturer of ROTARIX, for example,
there were sixty-eight (0.19 percent) deaths after administration of the vaccine in 36,755 individuals and fifty (0.15
percent) deaths following placebo administration in 34,454
individuals. Pneumonia was the most common cause of
death in both groups.

## CONCERNS AND CONTROVERSIES

In September 2010, the CDC stated on its Vaccines and Immunizations Web site that a safety monitoring study of ROTARIX vaccine conducted in Mexico by GlaxoSmithKline indicated that ROTARIX vaccine may cause intussusception in infants during the first week after they are administered their first dose. The CDC pointed out that if the risk for infants in the United States is similar to that seen in the Mexico study, it would mean 0 to 4 cases of intussusception from vaccine per 100,000 U.S. infants who received the first dose of ROTARIX.

The CDC noted that it still continues to recommend both the rotavirus vaccines—ROTARIX and RotaTeq—to prevent the disease. However, it also states that the findings of the Mexico study cannot rule out a risk of intussusception with RotaTeq that is similar to the risk regarding ROTARIX. Studies continue into the relationship between rotavirus vaccines and intussusception, and you can expect to see more study results in the future.

## LOOKING AHEAD

In November 2010, researchers from several universities, including Tufts, Boston, and Tulane, reported that they had developed a rotavirus vaccine that could be delivered as nasal drops and that had been tested successfully in mice. Even if subsequent research continues to see success, it will likely be a few more years before the vaccine is available for humans. In the meantime, scientists are also testing the nasal drop vaccine delivery system for tetanus, diphtheria, and pertussis.

# CHAPTER 5

## Diphtheria/Tetanus/Pertussis

Diphtheria, tetanus, and pertussis are three contagious diseases that can cause serious, life-threatening symptoms, which is why they are the targets of various vaccines designed for children, adolescents, and adults. The vaccine that is most often used to provide protection against these three conditions in children is the DTaP vaccine, but there are also other combination vaccines available for each of these three ailments.

Of these three diseases, the one that continues to present the biggest challenge in the United States is pertussis, also known as whooping cough. Despite the requirement from all fifty states that all children be vaccinated against these three conditions before they enter school, tens of thousands of cases of whooping cough are reported each year. Many of the cases occur in infants younger than 3 months old, and some of the infants die. One problem is that the vaccine cannot be given until infants are at least 6 weeks old. Even then, protection is not adequate until children receive a series of three shots.

The challenge of whooping cough is just one of the topics discussed in this chapter, where I will explore each of the three conditions separately, the various combination vaccines for children, and the newer vaccine for adolescents and adults.

## DIPHTHERIA

Diphtheria is a disease caused by the bacterium *Corynebacterium diphtheria,* which releases a toxin that is the factor responsible for a variety of symptoms that can range from mild to life threatening, especially in very young children. Until the diphtheria vaccine was first administered regularly in the United States in the early 1940s, tens of thousands of children and adolescents died each year from diphtheria. At one point, about 150,000 young people died in one year from the disease. Since initiation of the diphtheria vaccine, no more than five cases per year are diagnosed in the United States.

### Symptoms of Diphtheria

Symptoms of diphtheria usually first appear two to five days after a person comes into contact with the bacteria. The bacteria most often affect the nose and throat. The throat infection involves a gray to black covering that can block the airways. Not everyone who is infected experiences symptoms, but those who do may develop any number of the following:

- Bloody, watery discharge from the nose

- Bluish skin

- Breathing difficulties, such as trouble breathing, rapid breathing, or wheezing

- Chills

- Croup-like cough (sounds like a bark)

- Drooling

- Fever

- Hoarseness

- Painful swallowing

- Skin lesions

- Sore throat (may be severe)

Toxins released by the bacteria can spread throughout the body via the bloodstream and affect the organs, such as the heart and kidneys, and cause significant damage.

## How Diphtheria Is Transmitted

The bacteria that cause diphtheria can be spread through the air via droplets from a sneeze or cough of a person who is infected or from someone who carries the bacteria but has no symptoms. Diphtheria can also be transmitted via contaminated objects or foods, such as milk.

## Risk Factors for Diphtheria

The most significant risk factor for diphtheria is a lack of immunization. Others included living in crowded environments and practicing poor hygiene.

## Treatment in Infants and Children

Along with a physical examination of the throat, neck, and lymph glands, tests to diagnose diphtheria include a throat culture or Gram stain to identify *Corynebacterium diphtheria,* and an electrocardiogram (EKG). Because diphtheria can be life threatening, it is common to begin treatment even before test results come back. Immediate treatment includes diphtheria antitoxin administered in an injection or intravenously (IV), which neutralizes the diphtheria toxin in the body. Before being given the antitoxin, however, patients are usually given a skin allergy test to make sure they are not allergic to the antitoxin. If a child is allergic, he or she must first be desensitized to the antitoxin by slowly taking small doses of the antitoxin and increasing the dosage.

Antibiotics, such as penicillin or erythromycin, are the other treatment for diphtheria. Use of antibiotics can kill the bacteria causing diphtheria and reduce the length of time the patient is contagious. Children with diphtheria often need to be hospitalized and isolated in intensive care to avoid spreading the disease. In some cases, doctors remove the thick covering in the throat if it is making breathing difficult.

The death rate from diphtheria is 10 percent, and recovery is generally slow. Inflammation of the heart muscle (myocarditis) is the most common complication of the disease, although some patients also experience nervous system damage that may result in temporary paralysis.

## TETANUS

Tetanus, also known as lockjaw, is a disease that is caused by the toxin released by the bacterium called *Clostridiuim tetani*. When you think of tetanus, you may picture stepping on a rusty nail or cutting yourself with a dirty piece of glass, which are two ways the bacteria can enter the body and cause symptoms. Each year in the United States, about forty to sixty cases of tetanus are reported and about 30 percent of these individuals die. Death is more likely in newborns whose mothers have not been vaccinated and in patients older than 50.

### Symptoms of Tetanus

Once the bacteria enter the body, they release a toxin that causes the muscles to spasm. Muscle contractions can be so severe they can cause bones to fracture. If the spasms affect the throat and jaw (lockjaw), they can cause serious problems with breathing, resulting in suffocation. Other symptoms may include fever, sweating, elevated blood pressure, and rapid heart rate. The tetanus toxin can also damage heart muscle.

## How Tetanus Is Transmitted

The bacteria are found in the soil and in the intestinal tracts of animals and humans. These bacteria typically enter the body when you puncture your skin, as when you step on a nail or a piece of glass that is contaminated with tetanus bacteria. Contamination can also occur following burns, abrasions, and surgery. Tetanus is not spread from person to person.

## Tetanus and Pregnancy

What is the relationship between tetanus and pregnancy? A woman who has been immunized against tetanus passes the antibodies to her infant across the placenta. Women can become immune if they receive the vaccine before becoming pregnant or during pregnancy. If you plan to become pregnant or are pregnant and are uncertain about your tetanus immunization status or if your last tetanus shot was more than ten years ago, you should be immunized against tetanus.

It is important for expectant mothers to be immunized, as tetanus in newborns, once common in the United States, is prevented when the mother has been immunized. Women can get a vaccine that combines diphtheria toxoid and tetanus (Td vaccine) or a newer vaccine that also contains vaccine for pertussis for adults, Tdap. This vaccine has been licensed for use for women of childbearing age and can be given during pregnancy. The CDC recommends that pregnant women who were vaccinated with a tetanus toxoid-containing vaccine less than ten years ago receive Tdap post-partum according to the routine vaccination recommendations. (See "The DTP Schedules.") If their last dose of tetanus toxoid-containing vaccine was received more than ten years ago, the CDC recommends women be immunized with Td during their second and third trimester rather than receive Tdap.

## Treatment of Tetanus

Although there is no cure for tetanus, you can treat the symptoms and care for the wound. Proper cleaning of the wound helps to prevent growth of tetanus spores. Such cleaning can involve removing dirt and dead tissue from the wound. Several medications are also recommended. For example, the doctor may administer an antitoxin, which can neutralize any toxin that has not bonded to nerve tissue. Oral or injected antibiotics (e.g., metronidazole) are prescribed to fight tetanus bacteria, and a tetanus vaccine will be given to prevent future tetanus infections. Some patients need sedatives (e.g., diazepam) to control muscle spasms or medications such as magnesium sulfate or beta-blockers to help with heartbeat and breathing.

## PERTUSSIS

Pertussis, also known as whooping cough, is a highly contagious disease that makes children cough uncontrollably. The disease is caused by the bacterium *Bordetella pertussis* or *B. parapertussis* and typically lasts about six weeks. Pertussis is known as a toxin-mediated disease, which means the bacteria release toxins that are responsible for the symptoms. In this case, the bacteria attach to the hair-like structures (cilia) in the respiratory tract, produce toxins that paralyze the cilia, and cause the respiratory tract to become inflamed. The inflammation interferes with the body's ability to clear out secretions from the lungs.

Before introduction of a pertussis vaccine in the United States in the 1940s, pertussis was most common in infants and young children and, according to the CDC, more than two hundred thousand cases were reported each year.

Since the 1980s, however, the number of reported cases

of pertussis has been increasing, especially among infants younger than 6 months of age and among young people ages 10 to 19. More than thirteen thousand cases were reported in 2008, and many more cases are believed to have not been documented. In 2010, an outbreak of pertussis in California resulted in more than sixty-four hundred confirmed, suspected, or probable cases of pertussis in that state alone, most of which occurred in infants ages 3 to 6 months. This outbreak and others, including one in Australia, are discussed further under "Concerns and Controversies."

## Symptoms of Pertussis

The first symptoms of pertussis are similar to those of the common cold and usually appear about one week after exposure to the bacteria. Severe bouts of coughing (paroxysms) typically start about ten to twelve days later. The characteristic "whooping" sound at the end of a cough happens when patients try to take a breath but have difficulty because their windpipe is severely narrowed by mucus. The "whooping" sound rarely occurs in patients younger than 6 months of age and in adults.

Pertussis is also often accompanied by vomiting after coughing spells or a short loss of consciousness. Other symptoms may include slight fever (102°F or lower), runny nose, and diarrhea.

## How Pertussis Is Transmitted

Pertussis is an unusual disease because most children catch it from adults rather than from other children. The disease is transmitted when an infected person coughs or sneezes and minute droplets containing the bacteria travel through the air. Adults who have pertussis often do not know they have the disease and experience mild symptoms that are similar to a cold (remember, adults do not have the trademark "whooping" cough) and so they can easily spread the disease when they are around infants and young children.

## Pertussis in Infants and Young Children

Infants younger than 18 months who get pertussis should be monitored constantly because they may temporarily stop breathing when they have coughing bouts. In severe cases, infants should be hospitalized. Antibiotics such as erythromycin can be effective if started early enough, but they are less helpful if started later. Patients may need intravenous fluids if they are unable to drink enough fluids because of coughing spells. Young children may be given mild sedatives to help them sleep. Medications that should **not** be given include cough syrups, expectorants, and suppressants.

Infants and young children risk experiencing complications of pertussis, which may include pneumonia, convulsions, nosebleeds, permanent seizure disorder, ear infections, brain damage (due to lack of oxygen), cerebral hemorrhage (bleeding in the brain), mental retardation, apnea (slowed or stopped breathing), or death.

If there is a pertussis outbreak in your area and your child is younger than 7 years old and has not been immunized, he or she should not attend school or public gatherings and should be isolated from anyone known or thought to be infected. This isolation period should last until fourteen days after the last reported case in your school or other area.

## Treatment of Pertussis

Early treatment of infants and young children who have pertussis is essential to help prevent severe disease and life-threatening complications. If treatment is started during the first one to two weeks before coughing begins, symptoms can be reduced. A reasonable treatment guideline is to treat children older than 1 year old within three weeks of onset of cough and infants younger than 1 year within six weeks of cough onset. It is unclear whether giving antibiotics is beneficial for anyone who has been ill with whooping cough for longer than three to four weeks. Thus far, there are no effective treatments for the paroxysms of coughing characteristic of the disease.

If your child needs to be treated for pertussis, your healthcare provider will choose the best antibiotic course based on the possibility of adverse effects, drug interactions, and how well your child will tolerate the drug. Azithromycin is usually preferred for infants younger than 1 month of age, while erythromycin, clarithromycin, and azithromycin are preferred for children who are at least 1 month old.

## VACCINES FOR DIPHTHERIA, TETANUS, AND PERTUSSIS

The Centers for Disease Control and Prevention explain that there are four combination vaccines used to prevent diphtheria, tetanus, and pertussis:

- *DTaP:* the vaccine most often administered to children, it is for children younger than 7 years of age.

- *DT:* does not contain pertussis and is used as a substitute vaccine for DTaP for children who cannot tolerate pertussis vaccine.

- *Td:* a tetanus-diphtheria vaccine administered to adolescents and adults as a booster shot every ten years. Occasionally it is also given after someone has been exposed to tetanus.

- *Tdap:* similar to Td, but it also contains protection against pertussis. Adolescents ages 11 to 18 (but preferably at age 11 to 12) and adults ages 19 through 64 years should receive a single dose of Tdap. Adults age 65 and older who have close contact with an infant and who have not previously received Tdap should receive one dose. Tdap should also be

## HOW TO DECIPHER THE VACCINES

- Uppercase letters indicate full-strength doses of diphtheria (D) and tetanus (T) toxoids and pertussis (P) vaccine.

- Lowercase letters indicate reduced doses of diphtheria and pertussis, which are used in the adolescent/adult formulations.

- The *a* in "DTaP" and "Tdap" vaccines stands for "acellular," which means the pertussis component in the vaccine contains only a portion of the pertussis organism.

given to children ages 7 to 10 who are not fully immunized against pertussis.

A fifth vaccine, TT (tetanus alone), is also available for anyone who may have been exposed to tetanus (e.g., stepped on a nail or glass) and who is not current on his or her tetanus vaccinations.

### History of the DTaP Vaccine

In the mid-1940s, the tetanus toxoid vaccine was added to the vaccines for diphtheria and pertussis, creating the DTP vaccine. The DTP vaccine was used for nearly half a century, until the Food and Drug Administration licensed the DTaP vaccine in 1991 as an improvement over the original DTP vaccine.

The change in the vaccine was made because of side effects associated with the pertussis germ. Severe and sometimes fatal reactions were reported in about 1 in 140,000 cases of

DTP vaccine, which used whole cells of the pertussis germ. The DTaP vaccines use only small, purified pieces, which has resulted in fewer reported side effects. At first, DTaP was licensed to be given only as the fourth and fifth doses in the series, but in 1997 it was licensed for all five doses.

Overall, the DTaP vaccine is 95 percent effective in preventing diphtheria, tetanus, and pertussis. Specifically, it is nearly 100 percent effective in preventing tetanus, although the protection rates for diphtheria and pertussis are lower. The tetanus portion of the vaccine lasts only ten years, so the CDC recommends everyone get a booster dose of Td vaccine every ten years to maintain immunity.

## How the Vaccines Are Made

The bacteria that cause diphtheria produce a harmful protein called a toxin, so the goal of the diphtheria vaccine is to produce an immune response to the toxin in individuals who are immunized. To make the diphtheria vaccine, the toxin is inactivated with a chemical. This inactivated toxin is called a toxoid, and when it is injected into the body the toxoid causes an immune response to the toxin but does not cause the disease.

Similarly, the tetanus vaccine is made by taking the tetanus toxin and inactivating it with a chemical to create a toxoid, which is then injected into the body. The vaccine for pertussis has a slightly different story.

The bacteria that cause pertussis produce several different toxins, so makers of the vaccine select two to five of the toxins and inactivate them with a chemical. The version of the pertussis vaccine that is currently in use was released in autumn of 1996 and is called an "acellular" pertussis vaccine, which is designated by a small $a$ (e.g., DTaP). Before the acellular vaccine was available, the pertussis vaccine contained a killed form of the whole pertussis bacteria, or "whole-cell" vaccine. The whole-cell vaccine was associated with a higher rate of side effects, such as constant crying in 1 percent of doses and very high fever in one of every 330 doses. The newer, acellular form is purer than the old

## MORE ABOUT TOXOIDS

Unlike immunity that develops after your child receives a vaccination that contains a live, "weakened" virus, like that in the measles, mumps, and rubella vaccine or the chicken pox vaccine, the immunity that develops in response to inactivated toxins—like those in the tetanus and diphtheria vaccines—fades over time. That's why the American Academy of Pediatrics and the Centers for Disease Control and Prevention recommend that adolescents and adults should get the special formulation of the tetanus, diphtheria, and pertussis vaccine (Tdap) starting at age 11 or 12 and the tetanus-diphtheria boosters every ten years thereafter.

whole-cell vaccine and is associated with at least a tenfold less risk of side effects.

## The DTaP Vaccines

Before it's time for your child to get his or her DTaP vaccine, you should check the ingredients of each of the three main options, as well as consult your pediatrician about the risks and benefits for your child. The three current DTaP options are Daptacel, Infanrix, and Tripedia. All three are inactivated bacterial vaccines containing the same three microorganisms (*Bordetella pertussis, Corynebacterium diphtheria, Clostridium tetani*) and are administered via intramuscular injection at a standard dose of 0.5 milliliters.

A fourth option, Boostrix, is for anyone who has reached the age of 10 years or older and who has not been vaccinated for the three diseases. Also discussed here are two combination vaccines: Kinrix, which is for diphtheria, tetanus, pertussis, and polio; and Pediarix, which is designed for the same four diseases plus hepatitis B.

## Infanrix

Ingredients include aluminum hydroxide (no more than 0.625 mg), formaldehyde (no more than 100 mcg), polysorbate 80 (no more than 100 mcg), sodium chloride (4.5 mg /mL), and glutaraldehyde. Infanrix does not contain preservatives. Latex may be present in the tip cap and/or rubber plunger of the syringe.

## Daptacel

This vaccine contains aluminum phosphate (0.33 mg), formaldehyde (less than 0.1 mg), glutaraldehyde (no more than 50 nanograms), ammonium sulfate, and formalin. The preservative used is 2-phenoxyethanol (3.3 mg), and latex may be present in the stopper vial.

## Tripedia

The Tripedia vaccine contains aluminum potassium sulfate (no more than 0.17 mg), formaldehyde (no more than 100 mcg), gelatin, polysorbate 80, and ammonium sulfate. The preservative thimerosal is present (no more than 0.3 mcg), and latex may be present in the stopper vial.

## Boostrix

The Tdap vaccine (Boostrix) is recommended for all people 10 to 64 years old who have not previously received vaccinations against diphtheria, tetanus, or pertussis. The vaccine differs from the DTaP vaccine given to infants and young children because it contains a lesser amount of diphtheria and pertussus proteins and therefore is less likely than DTaP to cause side effects such as pain, tenderness, and redness in adolescents. Five years should pass between the time your child gets his or her last dose of the recommended DTaP series and the booster dose of Tdap, or between administration of the Td vaccine and administration of Tdap.

The Tdap vaccine contains the following ingredients: aluminum hydroxide (not more than 0.39 mg), formaldehyde (no more than 100 mcg), polysorbate 80 (no more than 100 mcg), sodium chloride (4.5 mg/mL), and glutaraldehyde. Latex may be present in the stopper vial. No preservatives are used to make Boostrix.

The two combination vaccines are described here.

## Kinrix

Kinrix (GlaxoSmithKline) is a vaccine whose diphtheria, tetanus, and pertussis components are the same as those in Infanrix and Pediarix (see later) and whose poliovirus component is the same as that in Pediarix. (See chapter 11 for more on polio.) A single dose of Kinrix can be used as the fifth dose in the DTaP vaccine series and as the fourth dose in the inactivated polio vaccine (IPV) series in children ages 4 through 6 years who have previously received Infanrix and/or Pediarix for the first three doses and Infanrix for the fourth dose. In addition to components for diphtheria, tetanus, pertussis, and polio, each 0.5 mL dose contains no more than 0.6 mg of aluminum hydroxide, 4.5 mg of sodium chloride, no more than 100 mcg each of formaldehyde and polysorbate 80, no more than 0.05 ng of neomycin, and no more than 0.01 ng of polymyxin B. Kinrix does not contain preservatives. Kinrix is available in two types of prefilled syringes, both of which have a tip cap that contains latex.

## Pediarix

Pediarix (GlaxoSmithKline) is a vaccine whose diphtheria, tetanus, and pertussis components are the same as those in Infanrix and whose hepatitis B antigen is the same as that in Engerix-B. (See chapter 3.) It also contains the antigens for the three types of poliovirus. (See chapter 11.)

Three doses of Pediarix make up a primary immunization course for diphtheria, tetanus, pertussis, and polio and the complete vaccination course for hepatitis B. Pediarix may be given to children as young as 6 weeks of age through 6 years of age. In addition to components for the five different diseases, each 0.5 mL dose contains not more than 0.85 mg aluminum salts, 4.5 mg of sodium chloride, no more than 100 mcg each of residual formaldehyde and polysorbate 80, no more than 0.05 ng of neomycin sulfate, no more than 0.01 ng of polymyxin B, and no more than 5 percent yeast protein. The two types of prefilled syringes used to administer Pediarix have tip caps that may contain latex.

## Who Should Get the DTP Vaccines

- Most infants and children younger than 7 years of age should receive DTaP beginning at age 2 months.

- Children younger than 7 years of age who cannot receive a pertussis-containing vaccine for some reason should be given the DT vaccine.

- Children ages 7 to 9 years of age can be given the Td vaccine as an initial catch-up immunization.

- All individuals age 7 years and older should receive the Td vaccine every ten years to provide continued immunity against diphtheria and tetanus and to help prevent tetanus for a tetanus-prone injury if more than five years have passed since the last dose of a tetanus toxoid-containing vaccine.

- Adolescents ages 10 to 18 years should receive a single dose of Tdap instead of a Td booster shot if they have finished the recommended childhood series of DTaP and have not received Td or Tdap. The preferred age to receive the Tdap vaccination is 11 to 12 years. Any child who has already received a Td booster should wait at least five years before getting the Tdap to reduce the chances of experiencing any local and systemic reactions.

- Adults ages 19 to 64 years should receive a single dose of Tdap to replace a single dose of Td for booster immunization if their most recent tetanus toxoid-containing vaccine was received ten or more years earlier. Adults can get Tdap at an interval shorter than ten years since their last tetanus toxoid-containing vaccine to protect against pertussis, especially if they are:
  - Women younger than 65 who are planning to become pregnant.
  - Men and women younger than 65 who have or who plan to have close contact with infants younger than 12 months. These adults should receive a single dose of Tdap and trivalent inactivated influenza vaccine (see chapter 6), ideally at least two weeks before contact with infants. These vaccines are important in this adult population because both pertussis and flu are easily transmitted to infants from adults.
  - Health-care personnel who have direct patient contact—including contact with infants and children. They should receive a single dose of Tdap.

All fifty states and the District of Columbia require vaccination for diphtheria, tetanus, and pertussis before children can enter school. See the Immunization Action Coalition entry in the appendices for links to specific information for each state.

## The DTP Schedules

- The DTaP vaccine is given in a series of five injections at ages 2, 4, 6, and 15 to 18 months and again at 4 to 6 years of age. If the fourth dose is given after a child is 4 years old, then no fifth dose is necessary.

- Any child younger than age 7 who is not able to receive the pertussis vaccine should be given the

DT vaccine. Between the ages of 7 and 9 years, he or she should be given the Td vaccine. This vaccine contains the same amount of tetanus vaccine as in DTaP or DT but less diphtheria toxoid.

- Any child age 7 to 9 years who has not been immunized should be given the Td vaccine instead of DTaP (or any combination vaccine that includes a pertussis element) because there are no pertussis-containing vaccines licensed for this age group. Two doses of Td should be given one to two months apart, and a third dose should be administered six to twelve months after the second dose.

- The Tdap vaccine should be given as a booster shot to children at age 11 to 12 (and no later than age 16 years). A booster of Td is needed every ten years thereafter to maintain protection against diphtheria and tetanus.

- Adults should receive a booster dose of Tdap to replace a Td booster. Thereafter a booster of Td is needed every ten years to protect against diphtheria and tetanus.

Parents should keep accurate records of their children's vaccinations, especially if the family moves and/or changes doctors and records may be lost or hard to locate. It is not unusual for children to be given combination vaccines from different manufacturers, but this can make the dosing schedule more complicated. Health-care professionals attempt to choose vaccines for children based on what they have already been given. Therefore, if you can provide accurate records to your doctor, you will be doing your children and your doctor a favor.

## OTHER VACCINES FOR DIPHTHERIA, TETANUS, AND/OR PERTUSSIS

(Including Manufacturer and License Date)

- Tetanus Toxoid (TT), Sanofi Pasteur, 1978

- Tetanus Toxoid Adsorbed (TT), Sanofi Pasteur, 1978

- Diphtheria and Tetanus Toxoids Adsorbed (DT), Sanofi Pasteur, 1984

- Tetanus and Diphtheria Toxoids Adsorbed for Adult Use (Td), Massachusetts Public Health Biologic Laboratories, 1970; Aventis Pasteur, 1978

- TriHIBit (DTaP and Hib conjugate vaccine), Sanofi Pasteur, 2001

- DECAVAC (TD; Tetanus and Diphtheria Toxoids Adsorbed for Adult Use, preservative-free), Sanofi Pasteur, 2004

- ADACEL (Tdap; Tetanus Toxoid, reduced diphtheria toxoid and acellular pertussis vaccine adsorbed), Sanofi Pasteur, 2005

- Pentacel (DTaP, Hib conjugate, hepatitis B, and inactivated polio vaccines), Sanofi Pasteur, 2008. This vaccine is not licensed for use in children older than 4 years of age.

## When to Delay or Avoid the DTP Vaccines

Some infants, children, and adolescents should not be given some or all of the vaccines for diphtheria, tetanus, and pertussis. Individuals who need to avoid such vaccines include the following:

- Anyone who has a history of a serious allergic reaction to any of the components of the vaccines should avoid them.

- Anyone who has a history of encephalopathy (e.g., prolonged seizures, coma) not attributable to an identifiable cause within seven days of receiving a vaccine that contains pertussis components.

- Children ages 7 to 9 years of age should not be given any vaccine that contains pertussis components.

- Tdap should not be given to anyone within two years after they have received a tetanus toxoid-containing vaccine.

- Anyone who developed Guillain-Barre syndrome within six weeks of receiving a tetanus shot should not get the DTaP vaccine.

If your child (or yourself or others) meets any of the following conditions, a health-care professional should be consulted before the DTaP vaccine is given:

- Has had a moderate or severe reaction after receiving a previous DTaP injection

- Has had seizures or having a parent or sibling who has had a seizures

- Brain condition that is unstable or getting worse

- Moderate or severe illness—any condition that is worse than a mild cold

## Side Effects of the DTP Vaccines

The DTaP vaccine may cause some mild side effects, including crankiness, decreased appetite, fever, soreness at the injection site, and vomiting, that typically last only a few days. Ask your health-care provider if you can give your child acetaminophen before and/or after the immunization to treat minor side effects. Frequently and gently moving the limb that received the injection can reduce the soreness.

Based on clinical trials by the manufacturer of the DTaP vaccine Infanrix, the occurrence of side effects is as follows. These figures are typical for all DTaP vaccines:

- Pain, redness, and swelling at the injection site: 10 percent to 53 percent of patients. These symptoms were highest after doses 4 and 5.

- Fever following doses 1, 2, and 3: 20 to 30 percent.

- Drowsiness, irritability/fussiness, loss of appetite: 15 to 60 percent depending on event and dose number.

On rare occasions, moderate to severe reactions have been known to occur. These may include nonstop crying for more than three hours (occurs in 1 in 1,000 children), fever higher than 105°F (1 in 16,000 children), or seizures (1 in 14,000 children).

Severe reactions to the DTaP vaccine are extremely rare, less than 1 per 1 million children. Such reactions include breathing difficulties, low blood pressure, and shock and occur within fifteen to thirty minutes of receiving the vaccine. Allergic reactions can be treated with medications.

## CONCERNS AND CONTROVERSIES

In 2010 and into 2011, the number of cases of pertussis reached record levels in the United States. From January 1 through December 31, 2010, in the state of California, for example, there were 9,477 cases of pertussis, including ten infant deaths. This was the most cases reported in sixty-five years, when 13,492 cases were reported in 1945. All of the deaths occurred in infants who were younger than 3 months old, and therein stir a few questions: One, since the first pertussis vaccine is administered at age 2 months or later, should the vaccine be given earlier? None of the vaccines currently on the market are for infants younger than 2 months of age. Or, because infants and children typically get pertussis from adults, is there a way to ensure adults are vaccinated against the disease so they don't pass it along to the young? In California, the state health department epidemiologists estimated that 50 percent of the children who got pertussis were infected by their parents or caregivers. The take-home message from the CDC: parents, grandparents, siblings, and others—including health-care professionals—who come into close contact with young babies should be vaccinated against pertussis. Unfortunately, the pertussis vaccine does not have a long life: it offers protection for only about five years, and then you need a booster shot.

# CHAPTER 6

*Haemophilus influenzae* Type B

In May 2011, the results of a national survey were released by the *New England Journal of Medicine* which reported that vaccination against bacteria that cause meningitis had led to a significant decline in cases of the deadly disease. One of the two vaccines credited with this improvement was Hib, which is used to fight *Haemophilus influenzae* type B, and the topic of this chapter. The other was a vaccine against *Streptococcus pneumonia,* which is covered in chapter 7.

The good news from the report is that the rate of bacterial meningitis declined by 55 percent in the United States in the early 1990s, when the Hib vaccine for infants was introduced.[1] The rates for bacterial meningitis continue to decline, especially in young children. However, when the disease does strike it often results in death.

Before the Hib vaccine was introduced in the United States, *H. influenzae* type B was the leading cause of bacterial meningitis among children younger than 5 years. The disease struck about twenty thousand young children each year, and for about one thousand it proved fatal. Today, however, the statistics are much more promising: an average of fewer than 1 in every 100,000 children develop Hib each year.

In this chapter I explore bacterial meningitis and the other diseases associated with Hib infection and the vaccines available to prevent them.

## WHAT IS *HAEMOPHILUS INFLUENZAE* TYPE B?

*H. influenzae* is a group of bacteria that can cause a variety of infections in infants, children, and adults. Overall there are six different types of *H. influenzae*, types a through f, but type-b organisms (Hib) are the ones that can cause serious invasive diseases early in life, which is why a vaccine was developed to protect infants and young children. (The vaccine is recommended for some adults as well.)

*H. influenzae* type b organisms make up 95 percent of all the six strains that cause invasive diseases. Although the name suggests *H. influenzae* causes flu, there is some disagreement over whether these bacteria can truly be said to cause flu, since influenza is traditionally caused by viruses. However, some experts say *H. influenzae* causes a type of flu caused by bacteria. In any case, these microorganisms are responsible for a number of infections, some life threatening, that can affect the brain, ears, eyes, lungs, and other parts of the body. Infants and young children are most affected by Hib, while cases among adults are rare. However, adults can be carriers and transmit the disease to youngsters as well.

### Symptoms of Hib Infection

The symptoms of an *H. influenzae* infection can mimic those of other conditions. In addition, symptoms can vary from child to child, even if they have the same condition. Therefore, it is best for a parent to consult his or her doctor to get an accurate diagnosis, especially if the child has not been immunized yet or has received only one or two doses in the series. Here are the conditions associated with Hib infection:

- *Middle ear infection*: Also known as otitis media, this ear infection may develop after a child has experienced a common cold. Symptoms may include tugging or pulling at one or both ears, difficulty sleeping or staying asleep, fever, fluid draining from the ear(s), ear pain, nausea and vomiting, diarrhea, congestion, loss of balance, hearing difficulties, and unusual irritability.

- *Conjunctivitis,* inflammation of the conjunctiva of the eye, which is the membrane that lines the inside of the eye and also the membrane that covers the eye itself. Symptoms may include redness, burning, and swelling of the eye(s), draining from one or both eyes, and hypersensitivity to light.

- *Sinusitis,* an infection of the sinuses that can affect younger children differently than older ones. Younger children tend to experience a runny nose that lasts longer than seven to ten days and have a discharge that is thick yellow or green, although it may be clear. They also tend to have swelling around the eyes, nighttime cough, and occasional daytime cough. Older children often complain of headache, facial discomfort, nasal drip, fever, sore throat, bad breath, and swelling around the eyes that is usually worse in the morning.

More serious conditions associated with type B include the following.

- *Meningitis,* an infection that affects the covering of the brain and spinal cord. Meningitis is the most common type of invasive Hib disease and represents 50 to 65 percent of cases. Symptoms of Hib meningitis in children older than 1 year include fever, stiff neck, back and/or neck pain, nausea and vomiting, headache, and reduced mental functioning. The condition can be difficult to identify in infants, who tend to have symptoms that include irritability, sleeping all the time, refusing a bottle, inconsolable crying, a bulging soft spot, and behavior changes. Between 2 and 5 percent of individuals who get Hib meningitis die, and 15 to 30 percent of survivors suffer some permanent neurologic damage, such as blindness, deafness, or mental retardation.

- *Pneumonia,* an infection of the lungs. It occurs in 15 percent of cases of Hib disease.

- *Epiglottitis,* a severe infection of the part of the throat that covers and protects the trachea and voice box during swallowing. The infection may cause fever, muffled voice, and rapid onset of a very sore throat. It can also cause swelling that results in life-threatening blockage of the airways. About 17 percent of all cases of invasive Hib disease cause epiglottitis.

- Infections that occur in less than 10 percent of cases include *joint infections* (septic arthritis), *skin infections* (cellulitis), *bone infections* (osteomyelitis), and *infection of the sac protecting the heart* (pericarditis).

## How *Haemophilus influenzae* Is Transmitted

The *H. influenzae* live in the upper respiratory tract and are transmitted from person to person either by direct contact or through droplets released by coughing, sneezing, or even having a close conversation. The infectious organisms enter victims through the nose and usually remain in the nose or throat, where they colonize and can remain for months without causing symptoms.

However, in some individuals the bacteria spread to the

lungs or bloodstream and cause invasive Hib disease. Infection can result in as little as a few days after exposure to the bacteria. Hib infections typically occur in children who have not completed their immunizations or in older children who did not receive the vaccine as infants.

Hib is an encapsulated strain of bacteria that have an outer layer composed of a polysaccharide called polyribosylribitol phosphate (PRP). The PRP is an important factor in determining how virulent the disease will be in any given person. You will see the acronym "PRP" as part of our discussion about Hib vaccines and perhaps during your own research as well.

## Risk Factors for Hib

The most important risk factor for Hib is contact with individuals who may carry the infection, typically in environments such as day-care settings and crowded households. American Indian and Alaska Native populations are also at increased risk for developing Hib disease, as are blacks who lack the Km(1) immunoglobulin allotype and Caucasians who lack the G2m(23) immunoglobulin allotype.

## Treatment of Hib

The typical treatment for Hib is a course of antibiotics for ten days, which may include ampicillin with chloramphenicol, cefotaxmine, or ceftriaxone. Most people who get Hib disease require hospitalization. Rifampin is used as a preventive treatment for people who have been exposed to Hib disease. Even with antibiotic treatment, 3 to 6 percent of children who contract Hib meningitis die from the disease.

## ABOUT THE HIB VACCINES

The first Hib vaccine was licensed in the United States in 1985. However, it was a pure polysaccharide vaccine, and therefore its ability to stimulate an immune response was highly dependent on age, and it was not very effective in children age 18 months and younger. Since the age group most susceptible to Hib disease is 18 months and younger, the vaccine was deemed ineffective and withdrawn from the market in 1988.

At the end of 1987, an improved Hib vaccine called a conjugate vaccine was introduced. The Hib conjugate vaccine is an inactivated vaccine that is made by chemically attaching a sugar (polysaccharide) to a protein, a combination that significantly increases the ability of the immune system in young children to recognize the polysaccharide and stimulate immunity.

All the licensed Hib vaccines are effective at producing immunity to invasive Hib disease, providing protection to more than 95 percent of infants after two or three doses. The vaccine will not, however, treat an active infection that has already developed in the body.

Since introduction of the Hib conjugate vaccine in the United States, the incidence of Hib disease in infants and young children has declined dramatically. The same cannot be said for infants and children in developing countries, where routine vaccination with Hib vaccine is not always available. This is one reason why children traveling to such countries need to take precautions. (See chapter 16, "Vaccines for Young Travelers.")

Even though the Hib vaccine is given to children to prevent disease, the number of Hib infections in adults has decreased as well. That's because far fewer children carry the infection and so they cannot infect adults.

Currently there are three Hib vaccines available that contain Hib alone, one that is combined with DTaP, and one in combination with recombinant hepatitis B vaccine. All the vaccines are administered via intramuscular injection. Here's a brief description of each vaccine. For simplicity's sake, the component *Haemophilus influenzae* type b capsular polysaccharide (polyribosylribitol phosphate) is referred to as PRP.

## ActHIB

ActHIB *Haemophilus* b conjugate vaccine (produced by Sanofi Pasteur SA) is licensed for infants and children ages 2 through 18 months. Each single 0.5 mL dose is formulated to contain 10 mcg of purified PRP conjugated to inactivated tetanus toxoid and 8.5 percent of sucrose. During manufacturing, ammonium sulfate, formalin, and formaldehyde (less than 0.5 mcg per dose) are involved in the process. The vaccine does not contain any preservatives.

## TriHIBit

When ActHIB vaccine is combined with Tripedia (see chapter 5), the result is the TriHIBit vaccine (Sanofi Pasteur SA), which is for children ages 15 to 18 months for prevention of Hib as well as diphtheria, tetanus, and pertussis. Each single dose (0.5 mL) is formulated to contain purified PRP plus antigens for pertussis and toxoids for diphtheria and tetanus, as well as 8.5 percent of sucrose. A trace amount of thimerosal (no more than 3 mcg per 0.5 mL dose) is in the vaccine from the manufacturing process.

## Hiberix

The Hiberix *Haemophilus* b conjugate vaccine (GlaxoSmithKline) is designed to be a booster dose for children ages 15 months through 4 years (before the fifth birthday) who have already received their initial Hib immunizations. In addition to PRP, each 0.5 mL dose is formulated to no more than 0.5 mcg of formaldehyde. The tip caps of the prefilled syringes may contain latex, although the plungers and vial stoppers do not. Hiberix does not contain preservatives.

## PedvaxHIB

The PedvaxHIB vaccine (made by Merck) is a PRP bound to a protein complex of a strain of *Neisseria meningitides.*

This binding is necessary to enhance the immune powers of the PRP. Substances used in the manufacturing process include ethanol, phenol, and enzymes. Each 0.5 mL dose of PedvaxHIB contains PRP and 125 mcg of the protein complex, as well as 225 mcg of amorphous aluminum hydroxyphosphate sulfate in 0.9 percent sodium chloride. No preservatives are used. The PedvaxHIB vaccine can be interchanged with other licensed Hib vaccines for the primary and booster doses.

## COMVAX

The COMVAX vaccine is a combination of Hib (Pedvax-HIB) and hepatitis B (Recombivax HB) and is manufactured by Merck. To produce the vaccine, the PRP is bound to the protein complex of *Neisseria meningitides* and hepatitis B surface antigen grown in yeast cultures that contain nicotinamide adenine dinucleotide, hemin, chloride, soy peptone, dextrose, amino acids, and mineral salts. Other substances used in the manufacturing process include ethanol and phenol. Each 0.5 mL dose of COMVAX is formulated to contain PRP, about 125 mcg of the protein complex, hepatitis B surface antigen, about 225 mcg of amorphous aluminum hydroxyphosphate sulfate, and 35 mcg of sodium borate. The vial stopper contains latex, and there are no preservatives in the vaccine.

Note: The HibTITER vaccine made by Wyeth (now Pfizer) has been discontinued.

## Who Should Get the Hib Vaccine

The following groups of infants, children, and adults should get the Hib vaccine:

- Infants and children beginning at age 2 months

- Adults and children who have sickle-cell disease

- Adults and children who have a weakened immune system related to cancer chemotherapy, HIV infection, or immunodeficiency

- Anyone who is HIV positive

- Anyone who has had their spleen removed

Parents should note that their children can get Hib disease more than once. Children younger than 24 months of age who have recovered from invasive Hib disease should be vaccinated as soon as possible.

The Hib vaccine is mandated in the District of Columbia and all fifty states except Delaware and Kansas. See the Immunization Action Coalition entry in the appendices for links to specific information for each state.

## The Hib Schedule

The recommended immunization schedule for Hib vaccine is:

- First injection at 2 months of age

- Second injection at 4 months of age

- Third injection at 6 months of age, unless your child received the PedvaxHIB or COMVAX brand of vaccine at 2 and 4 months, in which case the 6-month dose is not necessary

- Booster dose at 12 to 15 months of age

The injections given at 2, 4, and 6 months (if necessary) are called the primary series, while the injection at 12 to 15 months is the booster shot. It is important for infants and children to receive this vaccine on schedule because the diseases it is designed to protect against typically strike children between the ages of 2 months and 2 years. The shots in the primary series are not designed to provide lasting protection, so children need to get their booster shot as well before their fifth birthday.

Although the usual age for the first primary dose is 2 months, it can be given as young as 6 weeks of age. The recommended dosing interval for the first three (primary series) of vaccinations is 4 to 8 weeks. The fourth dose (booster) should be administered at approximately 12 to 15 weeks of age and at least two months after the third dose.

If the first two doses your child receives are PedvaxHIB or COMVAX and are given at age 11 months or younger, the third and final dose should be administered at age 12 through 15 months and at least eight weeks after the second dose. If your child's first dose is given at age 7 through 11 months, then the second dose should be given at least four weeks after and the final dose at age 12 through 15 months.

Dr. Bob Sears, pediatrician and author of *The Vaccine Book: Making the Right Decision for Your Child,* notes that there is one situation in which a child does not need to get the booster shot: if a child received his or her third dose at 15 months or later, the third dose is sufficient to protect the child, making the booster shot unnecessary.

The Hib shots can be given along with other shots. However, parents who are concerned about their child receiving multiple vaccines should discuss an alternative vaccination schedule with their physician.

## When to Delay or Avoid the Hib Vaccine

Situations in which children should not receive the vaccine or their dose should be delayed include the following:

- Children younger than 6 weeks of age should not be immunized.

- Any child who has had a severe reaction to Hib vaccine should not receive an additional dose.

- Children who are ill with a moderate or severe illness or who have a fever should not get the Hib vaccine until they are well.

- Any child older than 5 years who has not received the vaccine may not need to be immunized; discuss this option with your pediatrician.

As a side note, pregnant women should not get an Hib vaccination. It is not known whether the vaccine can harm the fetus.

## Side Effects of the Hib Vaccine

Your child may experience some mild side effects to the vaccine. The most common reactions are associated with the injection itself, such as redness, warmth, or swelling at the injection site, which occurs in 5 to 30 percent of children. Up to 5 percent of children develop a fever greater than 101°F. Less common side effects can include diarrhea, vomiting, and loss of appetite. In most cases, side effects resolve within forty-eight hours of the injection.

Some parents worry that the Hib vaccine may cause Hib disease. However, because the Hib vaccine consists of only a fraction of the Hib microbe, rather than the entire bacterium, it cannot cause disease.

## CONCERNS AND CONTROVERSIES

Similar to the hepatitis B vaccine, the first injection of the Hib vaccine is given at a very early age, which is a source of concern for some parents. Hepatitis B, however, is a disease that very rarely affects infants, while Hib diseases are most common among children ages 2 months to 2 years. Parents who are worried about their child receiving a vaccine at age 2 months should discuss their concerns with several health-care providers and fully understand the risks and benefits of the vaccine before making a decision.

Although cases of Hib disease have been very rare since introduction of the conjugated vaccine in the late 1980s, the disease has lifted its deadly head on several occasions over the years since then. In December 2007, Merck & Company recalled 1.2 million doses of Hib vaccine (PedvaxHIB and COMVAX) because of possible contamination with bacteria known to cause diarrhea and vomiting. The recall and subsequent halt in production of the two vaccines resulted in a vaccine shortage, which could be partly to blame for the rise in the number of cases of Hib disease. During January 2007 through October 2008 there were a total of 4,657 cases of invasive *H. influenzae* disease, of which 127 were type b and 2,263 were of unknown origin. Forty-five of the known Hib cases occurred in children younger than 5 years.

# CHAPTER 7

Pneumococcal Disease

In a report published in *The Lancet* in June 2011, experts noted that new technology in the development of vaccines had led to a significant reduction in complications and death due to pneumococcal pneumonia and meningitis, two potentially deadly conditions associated with pneumococcal disease. In fact, they pointed out that for pneumococcal disease alone, vaccination could prevent more than 1 million deaths per year worldwide caused by acute lower respiratory tract infections.[1]

Pneumococcal disease is a major cause of serious illness in children and adults around the world. It is caused by the *Streptococcus pneumonia* bacteria, and despite its name, the microorganisms are responsible for more than pneumonia. Currently, scientists are aware of more than ninety different pneumococcal types, and the ten most common types account for about 62 percent of invasive diseases worldwide. Fortunately, pneumococcal disease can be prevented with a vaccine.

The unfortunate news is that despite the availability of vaccines in the United States, thousands of infants and young children still fall victim to pneumococcal disease each year. According to unpublished data from the Centers for Disease

Control and Prevention (2009), an estimated forty-one hundred cases of invasive pneumococcal disease occurred among children younger than 5 years of age in 2008, and the thirteen serotypes that caused an estimated twenty-five hundred of the cases are those the current pneumococcal vaccine is designed to prevent.

What do you need to know about pneumococcal disease and the vaccine designed to prevent it? This chapter should bring you up to speed on the topic.

## WHAT IS PNEUMOCOCCAL DISEASE?

Pneumococcal disease is caused by *Streptococcus pneumonia,* bacteria that can attack many different parts of the body, resulting in a variety of conditions. Each of the following conditions can be the result of invasion by those microorganisms:

- *Community-acquired bacterial pneumonia,* which occurs when the bacteria invade the lungs. This type of pneumonia sends about 175,000 people to the hospital each year in the United States. Pneumococcal pneumonia is a common bacterial complication of flu and measles and results in death in 5 percent of patients.

- *Bacteremia,* which develops if the bacteria reach the bloodstream. More than fifty thousand cases of bacteremia occur each year in the United States, and about 20 percent of people who develop bacteremia die.

- *Meningitis,* which occurs when the bacteria attack the covering of the brain (meninges). About three to six thousand cases of meningitis occur annually, and one-third of people who develop meningitis die of the disease.

- *Otitis media* (middle ear infection), common in infants and young children, which develops if the bacteria reach the inner ear. More than 60 percent of children experience otitis media by 1 year of age and more than 90 percent of children by age 5 years. Although other bacteria can also cause middle ear infections, *S. pneumonia* is the one most commonly isolated from middle ear fluid. Before the childhood pneumococcal vaccine (Prevnar, discussed in this chapter) was introduced in the United States in 2000, the seven serotypes in the vaccine accounted for about 60 percent of cases of middle ear infection caused by *S. pneumonia*. Therefore, parents should note that while vaccinating their children with the pneumococcal vaccine will offer some protection against otitis media, there are other bacteria, for which there is no vaccine, that can cause middle ear infections.

- *Sinusitis,* which develops when the bacteria colonize the sinus and nasal passages.

Pneumococcal disease can affect people of any age, but those most susceptible include infants and young children, people 65 and older, anyone who has a weakened immune system, smokers, and individuals who have certain health conditions. (See "Risk Factors for Pneumococcal Disease.") The Centers for Disease Control and Prevention note that invasive pneumococcal disease causes more than six thousand deaths each year and more than 50 percent of these cases involve adults for whom vaccination against the disease is recommended.

## Symptoms of Pneumococcal Disease

The symptoms of pneumococcal disease depend on which infection develops. The four main types of pneumococcal disease and their symptoms follow:

- Pneumococcal pneumonia: chest pain, cough, fever, and shortness of breath

- Pneumococcal meningitis: disorientation and mental confusion, fever, photophobia (hypersensitivity to light), and stiff neck

- Pneumococcal bacteremia: chest pain, chills, fever, headache, joint pain, shortness of breath

- Otitis media: painful ear, red or swollen eardrum; sometimes fever, irritability, and sleeplessness

Infrequently, pneumococcal disease can lead to chronic problems, such as brain damage, limb loss, and hearing loss, and it can also be fatal.

## How Pneumococcal Disease Is Transmitted

The germs responsible for pneumococcal disease reside in the noses and throats of many people, and they are transmitted much like cold and flu germs are spread—through coughing, sneezing, and contact with respiratory secretions. Why these bacteria take hold in the body and cause disease is not fully understood.

## Risk Factors for Pneumococcal Disease

Although anyone can get pneumococcal disease, certain circumstances place some people at greater risk for the disease and its complications. The risk factors include:

- Age younger than 2 years or older than 65 years

- Having a compromised immune system due to cancer, Hodgkin's disease, human immunodeficiency virus (HIV), or leukemia

- Children who have a cochlear implant

- Presence of a chronic disease, such as alcoholism, diabetes, or heart, kidney, or lung disease

- Presence of sickle-cell disease or lack of a functioning spleen

- Being an Alaskan Native or member of certain American Indian tribes

- Being a resident of a long-term care or similar chronic-care facility

## Treatment of Pneumococcal Disease

Pneumococcal disease should be treated immediately with antibiotics, such as penicillin or a cephalosporin. The choice of antibiotic, how it will be given (orally or intravenously), and for how long will depend on which pneumococcal condition your child has, its severity, and your child's age. In recent years, there have been a growing number of reports of penicillin-resistant strains of pneumococcus in the United States, which means doctors must sometimes try several antibiotics before being successful.

## ABOUT THE PNEUMOCOCCAL VACCINES

Although pneumococcal infections can be treated with penicillin and other antibiotics, many strains of the disease have become resistant to these drugs. Pneumococcal infections affect highly susceptible populations, including infants and children; therefore, it is especially important to have an effective way to help prevent these infections. Thus three pneumococcal vaccines have been developed: two conjugate vaccines for infants and young children 2 years and younger, and a pneumococcal polysaccharide vaccine (PPSV) for adults. The polysaccharide vaccine is not used in young children because this age group does not respond to polysaccharide vaccines.

Children younger than 2 years of age, the elderly, and individuals who have certain chronic illnesses might not respond well, or at all, to the vaccine, while most healthy adults develop protection to most or all of the types of pneumococcal bacteria within two to three weeks of getting their injection.

Following are some details about the two pneumococcal vaccines on the market. A third vaccine for children, Prevnar, was discontinued as of October 1, 2010. Physicians who still have supplies of Prevnar (also sometimes referred to as Prevnar 7) may continue to use them: there is nothing wrong with the Prevnar vaccine, but it has been replaced with an improved vaccine called Prevnar 13. Infants and children who receive one or more injections of Prevnar should finish their series with Prevnar 13.

## Prevnar

Prevnar (Wyeth) is a pneumococcal conjugate vaccine (PCV7) that consists of antigens of *S. pneumonia* for seven serotypes (4, 6B, 9V, 14, 18C, 19F, and 23F). For this reason, Prevnar is called a 7-valent vaccine and is referred to as PCV7. Research shows that these seven serotypes are responsible for about 80 percent of cases of invasive pneumococcal disease in children younger than 6 years of age in the United States. The serotypes are grown in soy peptone broth and conjugated to diphtheria protein, which is grown in casamino acids and yeast extract. In addition to the serotypes, each 0.5 mL dose contains 0.125 mg of aluminum phosphate as an adjuvant. This vaccine is no longer being manufactured.

## Prevnar 13

Prevnar 13 (Wyeth; PCV13) was approved by the Food and Drug Administration (FDA) in February 2010 and supersedes

Prevnar (PCV7). PCV13 is approved for infants and children ages 6 weeks through 5 years (prior to the sixth birthday). It is a 13-valent pneumococcal conjugate vaccine, which means it consists of antigens for thirteen serotypes of *S. pneumonia* (1, 3, 4, 5, 6A, 6B, 7F, 9V, 14, 18C, 19A, 19F, and 23F) known to cause invasive disease. Prevnar 13 is also indicated for the prevention of middle ear infection (otitis media) caused by *S. pneumonia* serotypes 4, 6B, 9V, 14, 18C, 19F, and 23F. Currently there are no data available for serotypes 1, 3, 5, 6A, 7F, and 19A. The serotypes are grown in soy peptone broth and conjugated to diphtheria protein, which is grown in casamino acids and yeast extract. In addition to the thirteen serotypes, each 0.5 mL dose of the vaccine contains 100 mcg of polysorbate 80, 296 mcg of succinate buffer, and 125 mcg of aluminum phosphate adjuvant. The tip cap and rubber plunger of the prefilled syringe do not contain latex.

## Pneumovax 23

The Pneumovax 23 vaccine (Merck) is a pneumococcal polysaccharide vaccine designed for individuals age 2 years and older who have certain chronic medical conditions and/or who live in certain environments. Merck also recommends the vaccine for adults age 50 and older, while the CDC recommends adults age 65 and older be vaccinated. Pneumovax 23 consists of a mixture of highly purified capsular polysaccharides from twenty-three of the most common or invasive types of *S. pneumonia*, including the six serotypes that most often cause drug-resistant pneumococcal infections among children and adults in the United States. In addition to the polysaccharide mixture, each 0.5 mL dose contains 0.25 percent phenol as a preservative.

## Who Should Get the Pneumococcal Vaccine

The CDC has determined that the following infants, children, and adults should be vaccinated against pneumococcal disease:

- Infants and children younger than 2 years of age. Children who miss their shots or who start the series off schedule should still get the vaccine, although the number of doses and the intervals between doses will depend on the child's age when he or she gets the first shot.

- Healthy children 2 through 5 years who have not received any prior pneumococcal vaccinations or who have not completed the Prevnar 13 series should be given one dose.

- Children ages 24 months through 5 years who have any of the following medical conditions should be given one or two doses of Prevnar 13 if they have not already finished the four-dose series, or they can be given a dose of Pneumovax 23. The conditions include sickle-cell disease, a damaged spleen or no spleen, cochlear implants, leakage of cerebrospinal fluid, organ transplant, kidney failure, multiple myeloma, chronic heart or lung disease, asthma, or diseases that affect the immune system such as HIV/AIDS, diabetes, cancer, or liver disease. In addition, children who take medications that have an impact on the immune system, such as chemotherapy or steroids, are included in this group.

- Anyone ages 2 through 64 years who has a chronic health problem such as those listed immediately above, as well as people who smoke, should receive the Pneumovax 23 vaccine.

- All adults age 65 years and older should receive one dose of the Pneumovax 23 vaccine.

- Anyone who is a resident of a nursing home or long-term-care facility should receive the Pneumovax 23 vaccine.

PCV may be administered at the same time as other vaccines. If you are concerned about your child receiving multiple vaccines on the same day, consult your health-care provider about an alternative vaccination schedule. (Also see chapter 15, where I discuss alternative schedules.)

The pneumococcal vaccine is mandated for children in thirty-six states for entry into a day-care facility. See the appendices for the Immunization Action Coalition's Web site for information on the requirements in your state.

## The Pneumococcal Schedules

The CDC's Advisory Committee on Immunization Practices (ACIP) recommends the following dosing schedule for PCV13 for infants and children:

- First injection at 2 months of age, but can be given as early as age 6 weeks

- Second injection at 4 months of age

- Third injection at 6 months of age

- Booster injection at 12 to 15 months of age

If your child was born prematurely (less than thirty-seven weeks' gestation) and he or she is medically stable enough to receive vaccinations, PCV13 should be given at the recommended chronologic age along with other recommended vaccinations, according to the ACIP.

In addition to the basic vaccination schedule for pneumococcal vaccine, there are some alternatives based on whether your child started his or her series with PCV7, if your child started the pneumococcal vaccine series later than recommended, and/or if your child has a chronic medical condition. Naturally, you should discuss any options for your child's vaccination schedule with your pediatrician.

## Vaccination Schedule Alternatives

With that in mind, here are some of the alternatives you may need to consider. Discuss these options and variations with your health-care provider.

- Healthy children ages 7 to 59 months who have not been vaccinated with PCV7 or PCV13 previously should be given one to three doses of PCV13, depending on the child's age when vaccination begins and whether he or she has an underlying medical condition. Children aged 24 to 71 months who have an underlying medical condition should be given two doses of PCV13 at least eight weeks apart.

- Healthy unvaccinated children aged 24 to 59 months should be given one dose of PCV13.

- Children younger than 24 months who have received one or more doses of PCV7 should complete their vaccination series with PCV13.

- Children ages 12 to 23 months who have already been given three doses of PCV7 before age 12 months should receive one dose of PCV13, administered at least 8 weeks after their most recent dose of PCV7. The PCV13 dose will be the child's fourth and final PCV dose.

- Any child aged 12 to 23 months who has already received two to three doses of PCV7 before age 12 months and at least one dose of PCV13 at age 12 months or older does not need an additional dose of PCV13.

- Any healthy child aged 24 to 59 months who did not complete the PCV schedule with PCV7 or

PCV13 before age 24 months should receive one dose of PCV13.

- Any child aged 24 to 71 months who has an underlying medical condition and who received less than three doses of PCV7 or PCV13 before age 24 months should be given two doses of PCV13.

- Children older than 24 months who have underlying medical conditions and who already received three doses of PCV7 or PCV13 should be given a single dose of PCV13 through age 71 months.

- One supplemental dose of PCV13 is recommended for all children aged 14 to 59 months who have already received four doses of PCV7 or another age-appropriate, complete PCV7 schedule.

- Among children aged 6 to 18 years, those who have not received PCV13 previously and who are at increased risk for invasive pneumococcal disease because of various health conditions, such as HIV infection, cochlear implant, asplenia (no spleen), or sickle-cell disease, should be given a single dose of PCV13.

- Children aged 2 to 18 years who have an underlying medical condition should be given PPSV23 after they have completed all recommended doses of PCV13.

For children who are older than 6 months and who have not received Prevnar or Prevnar 13, the following catch-up schedule can be used based on their age:

- Ages 7 to 11 months of age: administer three doses, with the first two doses at least 4 weeks apart, and the third dose after the 1-year birthday, separated from the second dose by at least two months.

- Ages 12 to 23 months: administer two doses given at least two months apart.

- Age 24 months through 5 years (before sixth birthday): administer one dose.

## When to Delay or Avoid the Pneumococcal Vaccine

You should delay the pneumococcal vaccine if your child is ill with anything more serious than a mild cold at the time vaccination is due. Children who often get ear infections, sinus infections, or other upper respiratory conditions but who are otherwise generally healthy do not need to get the pneumococcal polysaccharide vaccine, because it is not effective against these infections.

## Side Effects of the Pneumococcal Vaccine

The most common side effects of pneumococcal vaccine in infants and young children are redness or swelling at the injection site, pain at the injection site, and fussiness. Fever and, rarely, febrile seizures have been reported in children as well. If your child is at higher risk of seizures than the general population, you can discuss alternative dosing with your pediatrician and/or the use of appropriate anti-fever medications your child may take around the time of vaccination to reduce the possibility he or she will experience fever post-vaccination.

To get a better idea of the side effects that occur with Prevnar 13, for example, we can look at the results of thirteen clinical trials in which about fifteen thousand doses were administered to 4,729 healthy children ages 6 weeks to 15 months who were inoculated using various three-dose schedules (at ages 2, 4, and 6 months; 2, 3, and 4 months; and 6, 10, and 14 weeks) along with a booster dose at 12 to 15 months.

The pneumococcal vaccine was delivered along with other recommended routine pediatric vaccines. A comparison group of 2,760 children received at least one dose of Prevnar 7.

Overall, at least 20 percent of children experienced injection-site reactions (pain, tenderness, swelling, redness), fever, decreased appetite, irritability, and a change in sleep (sleeping more or less) within seven days of each dose. These side effects were similar in both the Prevnar 13 and Prevnar 7 groups.

## CONCERNS AND CONTROVERSIES

Depending on which summary or review of the literature on pneumococcal vaccine you read, you will find different conclusions as to how effective the vaccine is in preventing pneumonia. For example, a Cochrane review of the research reported that healthy people who had received the vaccine were less likely to develop pneumococcal pneumonia than healthy people who did not get the vaccine. The reliability of this summary may be questionable because it included an older study that was not very high quality.

Another review evaluated slightly different studies and did not include the older low-quality study. That summary, published in the *Canadian Medical Association Journal,* suggested that the vaccine was not effective in preventing pneumonia, even for people for whom it was recommended, such as older people and anyone who had lung disease. This study, along with several others, has not made it clear whether the vaccine protects you if you are in poor health or if your immune system is weak.

It should be noted that the subjects of these studies were not children; they were adults, including some nursing home residents. However, the controversy has raised some concern among parents and guardians of children who have compromised immune systems or who have other conditions that put them at increased risk of developing pneumococcal disease.

# CHAPTER 8

Influenza

As every parent knows, influenza ("the flu") is often much more than a bad cold. Every year, parents everywhere brace themselves for the arrival of flu season and the bouts of fever, sniffling, coughing, aching muscles, and other symptoms that characterize the illness. For children, the flu poses a more dangerous health risk than the common cold, and it places a large burden on the health and well-being of children and their families.

Although you can always count on the seasonal flu to appear each year, you cannot count on the viral strains that cause the disease to be the same, nor the severity with which the disease will strike. Children younger than 5 years old typically require medical care when they get the flu. Every year, an average of twenty thousand children younger than 5 years of age need to be hospitalized because of complications associated with the flu, and those complications are most severe among children younger than 2 years old.

Infrequently, the flu presents a few surprises. During 2009–10, the world was hit by the first flu pandemic in more than four decades. The new, different flu virus was named 2009 H1N1, and it is estimated to have caused more than twelve thousand deaths in the United States alone. Unlike the seasonal flu, which is most lethal to people older than 65, nearly 90 percent of the H1N1 flu deaths occurred in people younger than 65.

The Centers for Disease Control and Prevention now recommend seasonal flu vaccinations beginning at age 6 months, with yearly shots thereafter. This chapter explains the disease the vaccine tries to prevent and the flu vaccines that are available for your children.

## WHAT IS INFLUENZA?

The flu is a contagious respiratory condition that is caused by influenza viruses. Flu is an unpredictable disease whose severity can vary widely from season to season depending on several factors, such as what flu viruses are involved, how much flu vaccine is available, when the vaccine is available, how many people get vaccinated, and how well the flu vaccine matches the flu viruses that are causing the disease in any specific season.

### Types of Flu Viruses

Influenza viruses are classified into three major groups—A, B, and C—and strains are further divided into various subtypes depending on the source of the virus and the types of proteins on the surface of the virus particles. Influenza A viruses are found in many animals, including birds, pigs, and humans. They appear worldwide, include H1N1, H1N2, and H3N2 viruses, and are the culprits in much of the severe illness during flu epidemics. The A viruses are also the ones that have a great ability to mutate rapidly and mix genetic material with flu viruses from other species of birds and mammals.

Influenza type B viruses circulate widely in humans. Although they have the potential to cause epidemics, mostly they produce a milder flu and are the viruses that typically cause children to miss school. Type-C viruses are found in dogs, pigs, and humans and cause mild respiratory infections but do not trigger epidemics. All influenza viruses change quickly as people become immune to the strains that are circulating in the environment. That's why the flu vaccine changes every year and your child should get vaccinated every year: because the immunity your child acquires one year will only partially protect him or her in subsequent years.

One thing parents can usually count on is a flu epidemic every year during the winter months, but an epidemic can extend into April and May as well. Young children are at great risk for developing serious complications associated with the flu, as are older adults, pregnant women, and anyone who has certain health problems, such as asthma, diabetes, or heart disease.

## Pandemic Influenza

A flu pandemic can occur when a new influenza A virus emerges against which people have no immunity and when the new virus spreads from person to person. The most recent flu pandemic occurred during the 2009–10 season when a new influenza virus that contained genetic material from swine, avian, and human flu viruses appeared. The virus was named pH1N1 2009, and it was responsible for a disproportionate number of illness and death among children, pregnant women, and people who had underlying health problems. The seasonal influenza vaccine for 2010–11 included this strain.

## Symptoms of Influenza

Uncomplicated cases of the flu generally appear suddenly, and symptoms can include any of the following: fever or feeling feverish and/or having chills, sore throat, cough, runny or stuffy nose, headache, muscle or body aches, fatigue, vomiting, and diarrhea. The latter two symptoms are more common in children than in adults. Symptoms can last for three to seven days, although your child may experience a cough for as long as two weeks.

The respiratory problems caused by flu viruses are difficult to distinguish from the illness caused by other respiratory infections. Young infants may experience symptoms similar to those associated with invasive bacterial infections and have a high fever and fussiness that require hospitalization. The majority of children hospitalized because of serious flu symptoms are less than 5 years of age, and most of them are released within a few days, although some need treatment in an intensive-care unit.

When flu attacks a child whose immune system is weak or compromised, complications can develop, such as bacterial pneumonia, dehydration, ear infections, and sinus infections. If your child has asthma, diabetes, or another chronic medical problem, having the flu can worsen his or her condition.

## How Influenza Viruses Are Transmitted

Flu viruses are spread primarily through the air in droplets when people sneeze, cough, or talk. The droplets take hold in the noses, throats, and mouths of people who are close by. Occasionally flu viruses can be transmitted if people touch surfaces or objects that have the flu virus on them and then touch their nose, eyes, or mouth.

Flu may also be transmitted by kissing or other close contact, so parents and other adults who are carrying the flu virus can transmit the virus to their children with a goodnight kiss or touching. Because most healthy adults can infect others beginning one day before they experience any symptoms, this can happen unintentionally. This is one reason why experts recommend parents and others who have close contact with children get the flu vaccine every year, to help prevent spread of the disease to children, especially infants who are too young to be vaccinated.

## Risk Factors for Influenza

Who is most likely to catch the flu and why? Experts have identified several risk factors of which parents should be mindful:

- *Age.* If you are the parent of a young child, you probably already know that seasonal flu tends to target young children, although it is also common among people older than 65. When the pandemic H1N1 virus appeared in 2009, however, it most often affected adolescents and young adults.

- *Living environment.* Children who live in close quarters at home, perhaps two or more siblings sharing a room, are more susceptible to developing the flu, as are children who live in dormitories at college or boarding schools.

- *Occupation.* Child-care workers and health-care workers are very likely to have close contact with individuals who are infected with the flu. Therefore, your child could be exposed to flu from any of these workers, including babysitters.

- *Compromised immune system.* Certain conditions can weaken your child's immune system, such as HIV/AIDS, cancer treatments, antirejection drugs, and corticosteroids.

- *Chronic illness.* Children who have chronic health problem such as asthma, diabetes, or heart disease are at greater risk of developing complications if they get the flu.

- *Pregnancy.* If you are pregnant, you are more likely to develop flu complications, especially during the second and third trimesters.

## Treatment of Flu for Infants and Children

Flu symptoms in infants and children may last more than seven days, but prompt care may slightly reduce the time your child isn't feeling well. Bed rest is essential, along with drinking lots of fluids, preferably water, herbal teas, and diluted fruit juices. Fever can be treated with acetaminophen or ibuprofen but never aspirin. Use of a humidifier in the child's room may help with breathing. Suctioning out the nose may be necessary, especially in younger infants. If your child has a dry or stuffy nose, saline nose drops may help loosen the mucus.

Currently there are four antiviral drugs for flu in the United States. If the drugs are taken within the first forty-eight hours of the onset of symptoms, the drugs may reduce the severity and duration of symptoms. One significant problem with these medications is that resistant viruses can slow your child's recovery. Another is that not all of them can be used in children, so you need to consult your doctor before starting treatment with any of the antivirals. Rimantadine, for example, is not approved for treatment of children younger than 13 years of age, while ribavirin (Rebetol) is for adults only.

Drugs called neuraminidase inhibitors are approved by the FDA for uncomplicated flu when the symptoms have been present for less than forty-eight hours. Zanamivir (Relenza) can be used to treat children older than 7 years of age, but it is not approved for prevention of flu. Oseltamivir (Tamiflu) can be given to children older than 1 year of age, is available in liquid, and usually must be taken for five days.

## ABOUT THE INFLUENZA VACCINES

One unique feature about seasonal flu vaccines is that they change year to year, depending on which viruses experts determine will be the most potent in the upcoming season. Each seasonal influenza vaccine contains three flu viruses: one A (H3N2) virus, one regular seasonal A (H1N1) virus, and one type-B virus. The three strains that will appear in any given year's flu vaccination program are selected by the World Health Organization Global Influenza Surveillance Network and are selected based on which ones experts believe are most likely to cause significant human suffering. The 2011–12 winter season flu vaccine, for example, was developed to protect against A/California/7/2009 (H1N1)–like virus; A/Perth/16/2009 (H3N2)–like virus; and B/Brisbane/60/2008–like virus, with the H1N1 strain being the same one used in the 2009 flu pandemic vaccine. The 2009 H1N1 vaccine was administered separately from the seasonal flu vaccine because the new viral strain appeared too late for it to be included in the 2009 seasonal flu vaccines. However, H1N1 was included in the 2010–11 seasonal flu vaccine.

Because flu viruses have a high mutation rate, a vaccine's formulation is effective for one year at most. Experts must make their choices many months ahead of the flu season so there is time for the vaccine manufacturers to prepare the vaccines. How effective are those vaccines? A 2008 study headed by Dr. David K. Shay reported that "full immunization against flu provided about a 75 percent effectiveness rate in preventing hospitalizations from influenza complications in the 2005–6 and 2006–7 influenza seasons."

According to the National Network for Immunization Information, when the match is close between the strains in the flu vaccine and the viruses that are circulating in a given year the flu vaccine can prevent illness in between 45 and 90 percent of healthy children.[3] Studies indicate that the vaccine is most effective in children who are older and healthier. The vaccination has also been shown to reduce middle ear infections among young children by about 30 percent.

## Types of Influenza Vaccines

There are two different types of flu vaccines, and each one is administered in a different way. Until 2003, all the flu vaccines on the market were trivalent inactivated (killed) influenza virus vaccines, or TIV, which are injected with a needle, usually into the arm. Prior to 2001, TIV was available in whole-virus and split-virus forms. Since 2001, however, only split-virus TIVs have been administered because they are associated with fewer side effects, including fever and injection-site reactions, than the whole-virus forms. The TIV is approved for anyone older than 6 months, including people who are healthy as well as those who have a chronic medical condition.

The newest type of TIV is a high-dose formulation (Fluzone High-Dose) introduced in 2010. This vaccine is only for people age 65 years and older. Older adults are advised to get a flu shot, not only for their own health but also to avoid passing along the flu to others, including young children.

In 2003, a new type of influenza virus vaccine was introduced: a live, attenuated, cold-adapted, temperature-sensitive, trivalent influenza virus vaccine (LAIV). The type A and B strains of flu virus in LAIVs multiply in the nasal passages but not in the lower respiratory tract. LAIV is available as a nasal spray and is approved for healthy individuals ages 2 to 49 years who are not pregnant. Children naturally prefer this flu vaccine because no shot is required.

Parents should note that flu vaccines are prepared using components from chickens and may cause an allergic reaction in children who have an egg allergy.

## AFLURIA

The AFLURIA vaccine (made by CS Limited) is a TIV licensed in 2007 for anyone aged 6 months and older. However, the ACIP recommended that the 2010–11 formulation not be administered to anyone younger than 9 years old because of "increased postmarketing reports of fever and febrile seizures in children predominantly below the age of 5 years as compared to previous years." This recommendation may or may not extend beyond the 2010–11 formulation.

AFLURIA is prepared from influenza virus propagated in fluid from chicken eggs. Therefore, if your child has an egg allergy he or she should not receive this vaccine. AFLURIA is formulated to contain 45 mcg hemagglutinin (HA; "hemagglutinin" refers to the ability of flu to "glue together" red blood cells) per 0.5 mL dose, with 15 mcg HA for each of the three influenza strains in the vaccine. Thimerosal is not used in the single-dose formulations, but multidose forms do contain 24.5 mcg of mercury per dose. Each 0.5 mL dose of AFLURIA also contains sodium chloride (4.1 mg), monobasic sodium phosphate (80 mcg), dibasic sodium phosphate (300 mcg), monobasic potassium phosphate (20 mcg), potassium chloride (20 mcg), and calcium chloride (1.5 mcg). The manufacturing process may also add residual amounts of sodium taurodeoxycholate (10 ppm), ovalbumin (egg protein) (1 mcg), neomycin sulfate (0.2 picograms [pg]), polymyxin B (0.03 pg), and beta-propiolactone (<25 nanograms). No latex is used in the rubber tip cap, plunger, or rubber stoppers.

## Agriflu

The Agriflu (Novartis, licensed 2009) vaccine is a TIV and is for individuals ages 18 years and older. The vaccine is prepared from flu viruses propagated in fluid from chicken eggs. In addition to the three chosen flu viruses, each 0.5 mL dose contains formaldehyde (no more than 10 mcg), polysorbate 80 (no more than 50 mcg), neomycin (no more than 0.02 mcg), and kanamycin (no more than 0.03 mcg. There may be latex in the syringe-tip cap. Agriflu does not contain thimerosal.

## Fluarix

The Fluarix vaccine (GlaxoSmithKline, licensed 2005) is a TIV available for individuals ages 3 years and older. Fluarix is prepared from flu viruses propagated in fluid from chicken eggs. Each 0.5 mL dose contains the three chosen flu viruses as well as octoxynol-10 (no more than 0.085 mg), alpha-tocopheryl hydrogen succinate (no more than 0.1 mg), polysorbate 80 (no more than 0.415 mg), as well as residual amounts of hydrocortisone (no more than 0.0016 mcg), gentamicin sulfate (no more than 0.15 mcg), ovalbumin (egg protein, no more than 0.05 mcg), formaldehyde (no more than 5 mcg), and sodium deoxycholate (no more than 50 mcg). The tip caps of the prefilled syringes may contain latex, although the rubber plungers do not. No thimerosal is used in the production of Fluarix.

## FluLaval

This TIV (ID Biomedical Corporation of Quebec, licensed 2006) is for people 18 years and older and is prepared using chicken eggs. Each 0.5 mL dose contains the three selected flu viruses as well as 25 mcg of mercury (from thimerosal), ovalbumin (no more than 1 mcg), formaldehyde (no more than 25 mcg), and sodium deoxycholate (no more than 50 mcg). No antibiotics are used to make FluLaval, and the vial stopper does not contain latex.

## FluMist

Licensed in 2003, FluMist (MedImmune Vaccines) is an LAIV for persons ages 2 through 49 years and is administered as a nasal spray rather than an injection. This vaccine is prepared using chicken egg fluid. Each 0.2 mL dose contains the three viruses as well as 0.188 mg of monosodium glutamate (MSG), 2.0 mg of hydrolyzed porcine (pig) gelatin, 2.42 mg of arginine, 13.68 mg of sucrose, 2.26 mg of dibasic potassium phosphate, 0.96 mg of monobasic potassium phosphate, and less than 0.015 mcg/mL of gentamicin sulfate. FluMist does not contain thimerosal.

## Fluvirin

Fluvirin (Novartis, licensed 1988) is a TIV for people ages 4 years and older. The vaccine is prepared from virus propagated in chicken egg fluid. Each 0.5 mL dose contains the three viruses as well as 25 mcg mercury (from thimerosal), residual amounts of egg proteins (no more than 1 mcg ovalbumin), polymyxin (no more than 3.75 mcg), neomycin (no more than 2.5 mcg), beta-propiolactone (no more than 0.5 mcg), and nonylphenolethoxylate (no more than 0.015 percent weight/volume). The tip caps of the prefilled syringes may contain latex, but the multidose vial stopper and syringe stopper do not contain latex.

**Fluzone**

Available for more than three decades, Fluzone (Sanofi Pasteur, licensed 1978) is a TIV for persons ages 6 months and older. The Fluzone High-Dose (2009) is for persons ages 65 years and older. Fluzone is prepared using chicken egg fluid. Each 0.5 mL dose contains the three recommended influenza virus strains plus no more than 100 mcg of formaldehyde, no more than 100 mcg of octylphenolethoxylate, and 0.05 percent gelatin. While the single doses do not contain mercury, the multidose forms contain 25 mcg of mercury from thimerosal.

The prefilled syringe tip caps of Fluzone may contain latex, but the vial presentation of Fluzone does not.

In May 2011, Sanofi Pasteur announced that it had received FDA approval for Fluzone Intradermal, a seasonal flu vaccine that is delivered via an ultra-fine needle that is 90 percent shorter than the typical needle used for shots. It is the first time such an ultra-fine needle has been approved in the United States for adults aged 18 through 64, although the needle has already been available in forty other countries. The new delivery system (microinjection) injects the vaccine into the dermal layer of the skin rather than into the muscle like traditional vaccines. Fluzone Intradermal contains no more than 20 mcg of formaldehyde, no more than 50 mcg of octylphenolethoxylate, no gelatin, and no mercury. There is no latex in this form of Fluzone.

## Who Should Get the Flu Vaccine

The Centers for Disease Control and Prevention recommend that everyone age 6 months and older get a seasonal flu vaccine each year. It is especially important that children younger than 5 years of age and children of any age who have a chronic health condition such as asthma, diabetes, heart disease, HIV, immune suppression, kidney disease, sickle-cell anemia, or any condition that can compromise lung function be vaccinated, as these children are at greatest risk of developing serious complications from the flu.

The CDC also recommends that people who have contact with certain groups of children also get a seasonal flu shot so they will not contract and pass along the flu to these children. Those people include:

- People who live with children younger than 5 years old (especially if they live with a child who is younger than 6 months old, because the child is too young to get vaccinated against flu)

- Caregivers of children younger than 5 years old (e.g., day-care providers, nannies)

- People who live with or who have close contact with any child of any age who has a chronic health condition

- Health-care workers

As of 2011, only two states—Connecticut and New Jersey—required children who are entering day care to receive the flu vaccine. See the Immunization Action Coalition entry in the appendices for links to specific information for each state.

## The Flu Schedule

For children who are receiving a seasonal flu vaccine for the first time, the CDC recommends the following:

- All children ages 6 months through 8 years should receive two doses of age-appropriate flu vaccine given four weeks apart.

- Children who received only one dose in their first year of vaccination should receive two doses in the following year.

- Two doses given four weeks apart are also recommended for children ages 2 to 8 years who are receiving LAIV for the first time.

- Vaccinations should begin as soon as vaccine is available and continue throughout the flu season.

- For healthy nonpregnant individuals ages 7 through 18 years, either LAIV or TIV may be administered.

Why do children need two doses? The first dose "primes" the child's immune system, while the second dose provides protection against the flu. If your child receives only one dose but needs two, he or she will have less or no protection from the flu viruses that year. Typically it takes about two weeks after the second dose for protection against the flu to begin.

## When to Delay or Avoid the Flu Vaccine

Some children and adults should delay or avoid getting immunized against the flu or avoid one of the two types of vaccines. Those people include the following:

- Infants younger than 6 months of age should not be immunized.

- Any child who is moderately or severely ill, including the presence of a fever, should delay getting the vaccine.

- Anyone who has experienced an anaphylactic reaction to eggs, egg products, or other ingredients in the flu vaccine should avoid getting immunized

- Children younger than 2 years of age and adults older than 49 years of age should not receive LAIV because the safety of this form has not been established in these age groups.

- Children ages 2 through 17 should not receive LAIV if they are taking aspirin or any medication that contains aspirin because the combination may trigger complications.

- Children and adults who have asthma or other reactive airway diseases should not be given LAIV.

- LAIV should not be administered to pregnant women, anyone who has a history of Guillain-Barre syndrome, or anyone who has a chronic underlying medical condition that may predispose him or her to severe flu infections.

- LAIV should not be administered concurrently with other live-virus vaccines.

## Side Effects of the Flu Vaccine

You may have heard that getting a flu shot causes the flu, yet because the vaccine contains killed viruses the vaccine itself cannot cause the flu. However, infants, children, and adults can experience side effects or reactions from flu shots, and reactions are more common the first time a child receives a flu shot. Common local flu shot reactions include soreness, pain, and swelling at the injection site, but these are typically mild and last for less than two days. Systemic flu shot reactions, which usually begin six to twelve hours after the flu shot is administered, can include fever, rash, muscle aches, irritability, drowsiness, and malaise (not feeling good). These symptoms usually last for only one or two days.

If your child is 2 years or older, he or she may be a candidate for the nasal spray type of flu vaccine (LAIV). Reactions to the nasal spray can include runny nose, nasal congestion, low-grade fever, headache, sore throat, muscle aches, tiredness, weakness, cough, chills, and sinusitis. Research shows that some children may experience an increased rate of wheezing after getting LAIV. If your child has experienced wheezing within the past year, then he or she likely should get a flu shot instead. Talk to your pediatrician.

In very rare cases, serious reactions can occur. If your child is allergic to eggs or to any other component of the flu vaccine, he or she may experience a severe allergic reaction that includes hives, swollen tongue or lips, difficulty breathing, and collapse. An extremely rare chance (1 per million) of developing Guillain-Barre syndrome, a progressive nervous system disorder, is associated with TIV. Any child who has a history of Guillain-Barre syndrome should not be given LAIV because its safety regarding this disease has not been investigated.

## CONCERNS AND CONTROVERSIES

In January 2011, the Food and Drug Administration and the Centers for Disease Control and Prevention announced they had recently detected an increase in the number of reports to the VAERS (the Vaccine Adverse Event Reporting System; see chapter 14) concerning febrile seizures (seizures related to a fever) in children after they had received the TIV Fluzone. Most of the seizures were reported in children younger than 2 years of age. Among the reported cases, all the children recovered without any lasting effects.

At the time of the announcement, investigations were underway to determine if there was an association between the flu vaccine and the febrile seizures or if other factors were involved. There was no increase in VAERS reports concerning febrile seizures in children older than 2 years of age after vaccination with TIV. At the time, the FDA and CDC did not change the recommendations for use of the flu vaccine in children. A shift in immunization recommendations, however, is always a possibility.

# CHAPTER 9

Measles/Mumps/Rubella

Measles, mumps, and rubella (German measles), commonly referred to as MMR, are the diseases covered in the MMR combination vaccine. Yet some of today's young parents may not realize that this trio of vaccines is not how children were first protected against these infectious diseases. Initially children received an individual shot for each of these diseases until the combination vaccine was developed. Today, parents who vaccinate their children against any of these infectious diseases must get the combination vaccine, as the individual vaccines are not available.

The MMR vaccine also is probably the vaccine that has generated the most controversy and media attention in recent years. I am of course referring to the proposed association between the MMR vaccine and autism, a link that was later proclaimed by medical experts to not exist. Some parents and other concerned individuals, however, believe the relationship *does* exist.

This chapter explores each of the three diseases covered by the MMR vaccine and the vaccine itself.

## WHAT IS MEASLES?

Measles, also called rubeola (not to be confused with rubella), is a highly contagious disease that is caused by a virus. Before a measles vaccine was available in the 1960s, more than five hundred thousand cases of measles were reported every year in the United States. In fact, nearly everyone in the United States got the measles by age 20. Although the MMR vaccine has largely eliminated measles in the United States, several dozen cases still occur each year. From 2000 to 2007, for example, an average of sixty-three cases per year were reported to the Centers for Disease Control and Prevention.

In some years, however, the number of cases is higher. In 2008, for example, a total of 140 cases were reported; more than 75 percent of the cases were linked to measles that had entered the United States from another country, and more than 90 percent of the people infected either had not been immunized or their immunization status was not known. In May 2011, the CDC noted that ninety-eight cases had already been reported for the year.

Around the world, about 20 million cases of measles still develop each year. Although the death rates have been falling worldwide, measles still kills several hundred thousand people per year, most of whom are younger than age 5 years.

### Symptoms of Measles

Hopefully you and your child will never experience the telltale signs and symptoms of measles, which is probably most recognized by the full-body pink/red rash it causes. The first symptoms, however, are typically a runny nose, high fever, red eyes (conjunctivitis), and a hacking cough. Also look inside the mouth for Koplik's spots, which are small red spots that have a blue-white center. The body rash usually first appears on the forehead and then spreads down the body.

Common complications of measles include middle ear

infections, pneumonia, croup, and diarrhea. An infection of the brain (measles encephalitis) occurs in 1 per 1,000 cases of natural measles and in some cases causes permanent brain damage among those who survive. About 5 percent of children who have measles also develop pneumonia.

A rare and fatal complication of measles is subacute sclerosing panencephalitis (SSPE). One risk factor for developing SSPE is getting measles at a young age. SSPE occurs in 7 to 11 cases per 100,000 cases of measles. What is unusual about SSPE is that symptoms of brain damage usually do not begin until seven to ten years after infection and death typically takes place one to three years after symptoms appear.

The death rate among children who get measles in the United States is 1 to 3 of every 1,000 cases. Death is more common among infants, malnourished children, and those who are immunocompromised with diseases such as leukemia or HIV.

## How Measles Is Transmitted

If your child has not been vaccinated for measles, he or she has a 90 percent chance of developing the disease if exposed to an infected person. People with measles are contagious from one to two days before they experience any symptoms and until about four days after their rash appears. The disease is spread when someone comes in direct contact with the infected droplets or when an infected individual sneezes, coughs, or talks and projects virus droplets through the air. It is also possible to contract measles from a surface upon which infected droplets have landed. These droplets can remain active and contagious for several hours, and children who touch a contaminated surface and put their fingers into their mouth or nose or rub their eyes can become infected.

## Risk Factors for Measles

Infants are usually protected against contracting measles for six months after they are born because they have immunity passed on to them from their mothers. After that time, the risk of infection increases. Risk factors for measles include:

- *Lack of vaccination.* Infants and children who are not vaccinated run the risk of contracting the disease from someone who is infected, including individuals who come to the United States from other countries.

- *International travel.* Unvaccinated individuals who travel to developing countries where measles is common are at greater risk of catching the disease. (Also see chapter 16, "Vaccines for Young Travelers").

- *Vitamin A deficiency.* A lack of sufficient vitamin A in the diet can make your children more likely to get measles and to experience more severe symptoms.

## Treatment of Measles

Because measles is caused by a virus, there are no specific treatments for the disease, including antibiotics. Therefore, parents must let the disease run its course, although you can treat symptoms. It is important, however, that you take your child to a doctor for a firm diagnosis, both for your child's sake and so your doctor can report the case to the authorities. Any child who contracts measles should drink plenty of fluids, get lots of rest, and be kept away from others to avoid spreading the infection. Supplementation with vitamin A may be helpful for children between 6 months and 2 years who are hospitalized with measles and its complications.

## WHAT IS MUMPS?

Mumps is an infectious viral disease that usually spreads through saliva and most often affects the parotid salivary glands, which are located between the ear and the ascending branch of the lower jaw. When these glands swell, it gives people with mumps the characteristic "puffed-up" cheeks and neck. The mumps virus is not confined to the salivary glands, however, as the virus can impact other parts of the body as well.

Before a vaccine for mumps was introduced in 1967, more than two hundred thousand cases occurred in the United States each year. Now fewer than one thousand cases are reported each year and epidemics are fairly rare. Before a vaccine was introduced, mumps mostly affected children ages 5 to 14, and this still holds true today, although the proportion of young adults who contract the disease has been increasing slowly over the past few decades.

## Symptoms of Mumps

Before the telltale puffed cheeks appear, mumps may start with a fever of up to 103°F, loss of appetite, and headache. The parotid glands become increasingly swollen and painful over about one to three days, and your child will have difficulty swallowing, talking, chewing, and drinking. The parotid glands on one or both sides may be affected, and if both sides are impacted the swelling may not occur at the same time. Children usually recover from mumps in about ten to twelve days, and it takes about one week for the swelling to go away in each parotid gland. Doctors believe that about one-third of people who have the mumps do not experience any symptoms.

Rarely, mumps affects the other salivary glands, in which case your child will likely have swelling under the tongue, under the jaw, or in the front of the chest. Rare complications of mumps include inflammation and swelling of the brain (encephalitis), the lining of the brain and spinal cord (meningitis), and other organs. Symptoms of these conditions usually appear in the first week after the parotid glands begin to swell and may include high fever, stiff neck, drowsiness, convulsions, headache, and nausea and vomiting.

A rare complication of mumps among male adolescents

and young adults is orchitis, which is inflammation of the testicles. Orchitis usually affects one testicle, although infrequently it affects both. One or both testicles becomes painful and swollen about seven to ten days after the parotid glands swell. Other symptoms of orchitis include high fever, chills, nausea, vomiting, headache, and abdominal pain that can mimic appendicitis if a boy's right testicle is affected. The symptoms generally subside after three to seven days.

One-third of boys who develop mumps will develop orchitis and end up with testicular atrophy, or shrunken testicles. In rare cases, sterility is a complication of orchitis.

In females, mumps may affect the ovaries, causing tenderness and pain in the abdomen. Mumps may also affect the pancreas in both males and females.

If your child does get the mumps, chances are very slim he or she will ever get the disease again because one bout nearly always provides lifelong protection.

## How Mumps Is Transmitted

The mumps virus can be spread both through the air via droplets and by touching surfaces or objects that have been contaminated by an infected person. Therefore, your child may contract mumps if an infected individual sneezes, coughs, laughs, or speaks within close distance. The virus can also be spread if your child uses a drinking glass or eating utensil from someone with the virus.

People who have mumps are most contagious from two days before they experience symptoms until about six days after they end. Even if an infected person does not have symptoms, he or she can spread the disease.

## Risk Factors for Mumps

If you are a mother who was immune to the mumps virus before you got pregnant (as most mothers are), then your infant received temporary immunity from you through the placenta. That immunity is good for six months and perhaps as long as eighteen months, although it declines over that time period. With that in mind, the risk factors for mumps include:

- *Age.* Although mumps can occur at any age, it most often affects children ages 2 through 12.

- *Exposure to the virus.* Anyone who has been exposed to unvaccinated people or to someone who has the mumps is at greater risk of developing the infection.

- *Immune system.* A weakened immune system places people at increased risk of developing mumps, even if they have been vaccinated for the disease.

- *Time of year.* People are more likely to get mumps in winter and spring.

- *Travel.* Although mumps does occur in the United States, it is much more common in other parts of the world. If your child will be traveling outside the United States, he or she should be vaccinated for mumps. (also see chapter 16, "Vaccines for Young Travelers").

## Treatment of Mumps

If you believe your child has mumps, contact your doctor immediately and get a firm diagnosis. This is important for two reasons: you and your doctor will need to monitor your child and watch for complications, and your doctor must report the case to health officials.

Because mumps is a viral disease, antibiotics are ineffective. However, you can treat and relieve the symptoms by using **nonaspirin** fever medications such as ibuprofen or acetaminophen. (Children who have a viral infection should not be given aspirin because the drug may cause Reye's syndrome, a condition that can lead to liver failure and death.) If the mumps involve the testicles, your doctor may prescribe a stronger medication for the pain and swelling.

You can also relieve your child's symptoms by applying warm or cold packs to the swollen glands, providing a soft, bland diet that does not require much chewing, and encouraging your child to drink lots of water, decaffeinated soft drinks, or tea. Avoid acidic fruit juices because they can make parotid pain worse.

## WHAT IS RUBELLA?

Rubella, or German measles, is a viral infection that mostly affects the lymph nodes and skin. Also known as three-day measles, rubella is not caused by the same virus that causes measles and is usually a mild disease in children. The main health concern about rubella, however, is among pregnant women, who can pass along the infection to their unborn child and cause congenital rubella syndrome. (See "Congenital Rubella Syndrome.")

Before the rubella vaccine became available in 1969, epidemics of the disease occurred every six to nine years and most of the children affected were ages 5 to 9 years old. Once vaccination of children was introduced, the number of rubella cases declined dramatically. Only about thirty to sixty cases of rubella are reported each year in the United States. Today, rubella appears more often among young, nonimmunized adults than among children. An estimated 10 percent of young adults are believed to be susceptible to the disease, which means anyone who becomes infected, especially pregnant women, could pass the virus along to unprotected children.

### Symptoms and Complications of Rubella

Once a child is exposed to rubella, the incubation period is fourteen to twenty-three days. The first symptoms of rubella are usually a mild fever and swollen, tender lymph nodes usually behind the ears or in the back of the neck. These symptoms last for about one to two days before an itchy rash appears on the face and spreads down the body. The rash is either pink or light red spots that may blend together to form colored patches. As the rash spreads over the body it typically fades from the face. After about three days the rash clears and the skin sheds fine flakes.

Teens and adults are more likely than young children to also experience headache, loss of appetite, conjunctivitis (pinkeye), painful swollen joints, and a stuffy or runny nose. Many people who contract rubella have few or no symptoms. If a woman contracts rubella during pregnancy, there is a risk of miscarriage or stillbirth or her child may be born with birth defects. (See "Congenital Rubella Syndrome.")

## Congenital Rubella Syndrome

Congenital rubella is caused by the rubella virus when it attacks the fetus during a critical time of development—the first trimester of pregnancy. Rubella after the fourth month is less likely to harm the developing child. However, any pregnant woman who has not been vaccinated and who has never had rubella risks damaging her unborn baby.

Women who plan to get pregnant should be vaccinated at least twenty-eight days before they conceive. Because the MMR vaccine contains a live virus for rubella, women who are pregnant should not get the vaccine.

Fortunately, fewer than five infants per year are diagnosed with congenital rubella syndrome in the United States. Signs and symptoms of the disease in infants include cloudy corneas, deafness, developmental delay, excessive sleepiness, irritability, low birth weight, mental retardation, seizures, small head size, and rash present at birth. There is no specific treatment for the disease, and nervous system damage is permanent. Complications may develop, including cataracts or glaucoma, heart defects, and bone disease.

## How Rubella Is Transmitted

The rubella virus can be transmitted from person to person via droplets of contaminated fluid from the throat and nose when people cough, sneeze, laugh, or talk. Anyone who has rubella is contagious from one week before to one week after his or her rash appears. Not everyone who develops rubella has symptoms, however, but they can still transmit the virus.

Infants who have congenital rubella syndrome can pass along the virus in fluid from their nose and throat as well as in their urine for up to a year or longer and infect people who have not been vaccinated.

## Risk Factors for Rubella

Risk factors for rubella include:

- Exposure to an infected person

- Not being vaccinated

## Treatment of Rubella

Children who get rubella typically experience mild symptoms. There is no specific treatment for rubella, and because it is a virus antibiotics are not effective. However, you can relieve symptoms by giving your child acetaminophen or ibuprofen. Never give your child aspirin for a viral infection because the drug may cause Reye's syndrome, which can lead to liver failure and death. If there are no complications, rubella typically resolves on its own within a few days.

## ABOUT THE MMR VACCINE

The MMR vaccine that parents are familiar with today did not start out as a trio. The first measles vaccines—both a live and an inactivated form—were marketed in 1963, but the two vaccines were mostly replaced by an improved attenuated live-virus vaccine that was licensed in 1968. A vaccine for mumps made its debut in 1967, and a rubella vaccine followed in 1969. In 1971, the three vaccines were combined into one to form the MMR vaccine. In 2005, a vaccine that combines both MMR and chicken-pox (varicella) vaccines, known as MMRV, was introduced to the market. As of 2010, single vaccines for measles (Attenuvax), mumps (Mumpsvax), and rubella (Meruvax) were no longer available in the United States.

When the MMR vaccine was first developed, only one dose was given and it was effective in 90 to 95 percent of children. Then, in 1989, the American Academy of Pediatrics, the American Academy of Family Physicians, and the Centers for Disease Control and Prevention's Advisory Committee on Immunization Practices changed the recommendation to include two doses, which meant that 99.7 percent of children would be protected.

## Types of MMR Vaccines

As of 2011, only two vaccines were available to help prevent measles, mumps, and rubella, and one of the two is also for varicella.

### M-M-R II
The M-M-R II (licensed 1971, made by Merck) is a live vaccine that consists of preparations of Attenuvax, Mumpsvax, and Meruvax II. Both Attenuvax and Mumpsvax are produced in chick embryo cell culture, and Meruvax II is prepared in human lung cells. Each 0.5 mL dose contains 14.5 mg of sorbitol, 1.9 mg of sucrose, 14.5 mg of hydrolyzed gelatin, no more than 0.3 mg of recombinant human albumin, less than 1 ppm of fetal bovine serum, approximately 25 mcg of neomycin, as well as sodium phosphate, sodium chloride, and other buffer and media ingredients. M-M-R II contains no preservatives.

## ProQuad

The ProQuad vaccine (licensed 2005, made by Merck) is a combined, attenuated, live vaccine that is designed to prevent measles, mumps, rubella, and varicella (chicken pox). It contains components of the M-M-R II vaccine (which means two of the strains were prepared using chick embryo cell culture) along with the varicella virus vaccine live prepared in human lung tissue culture. Each 0.5 mL dose of ProQuad contains no more than 21 mg of sucrose, 11 mg of hydrolyzed gelatin, 2.4 mg of sodium chloride, 1.8 mg of sorbitol, 0.40 mg of monosodium glutamate, 0.34 mg of sodium phosphate dibasic, 0.31 mg of human albumin, 0.17 mg of sodium bicarbonate, 72 mcg of potassium phosphate monobasic, 60 mcg of potassium chloride, 36 mcg of potassium phosphate dibasic, less than 16 mcg of neomycin, 0.5 mcg of bovine calf serum, and other buffer and media ingredients. There are no preservatives in ProQuad.

## Who Should Get the MMR Vaccine

The CDC recommends the following individuals get the MMR vaccine:

- Individuals age 12 months and older.

- Anyone age 18 years or older who was born after 1956, unless they can show they have had either the vaccines or the diseases. Adults born during or before 1956 are believed to be immune.

- Women who are of reproductive age and who have not received the MMR vaccination should have a blood test to see if they are immune. If they are not, they should get the vaccine, but not if they are pregnant or planning to get pregnant within the next one to three months, because it may harm the baby.

All fifty states and the District of Columbia mandate the MMR vaccine for children before they enter school. See the Immunization Action Coalition entry in the appendices for links to specific information for each state.

## The MMR Schedule

The recommended vaccination schedule for MMR is:

- First shot at 12 to 15 months of age

- Booster shot at 4 to 6 years of age

As always, there are exceptions to the rule. If there is an outbreak of measles, mumps, or rubella and your child is between the ages of 6 and 11 months old, he or she can be given the MMR vaccine. However, this should be followed by another shot at 12 to 15 months and again at 4 to 6 years of age. Similarly, if there is an outbreak of any of the three diseases and your child is between 1 and 4 years old your doctor may recommend an additional shot.

If there is an outbreak of measles and your child has not been immunized, especially if he or she has a weakened immune system, your doctor can help protect your child from measles with an injection of measles antibodies called immune globulin if it is given within six days of exposure. The antibodies can either prevent measles or make the symptoms less severe. The measles vaccine may also protect your child against measles, but it must be given within seventy-two hours of exposure to the disease.

The CDC's catch-up vaccination schedule can be seen in the appendices.

## Who Should Delay or Avoid the MMR Vaccine

Not every child is a candidate for an MMR vaccination. For example, the vaccine should be delayed or avoided in the following cases:

- Children who are experiencing any illness more serious than a mild cold should delay receiving the vaccine.

- Children and others who have untreated tuberculosis, leukemia, or other cancers or whose immune systems are compromised for any reason should not be given the vaccine.

- Children and others who have a history of severe allergic reaction to gelatin, chicken eggs, or the antibiotic neomycin should not get the MMR vaccine, because these ingredients can cause serious reactions.

- Children and others who are receiving blood products (except washed red blood cells) such as immune globulin should delay receiving the MMR vaccine for 3 to 11 months, depending on which blood product they are getting and the dosage.

- Women who are pregnant or who are trying to get pregnant should not get the vaccine. In addition, women should not become pregnant within twenty-eight days after getting immunized with MMR.

## What to Know About ProQuad

ProQuad is the vaccine that combines MMR plus varicella (the vaccine for chicken pox). Because the MMR and varicella vaccines are scheduled to be given during the same time range, some parents choose to have their child receive one injection (ProQuad) instead of two (individual M-M-R II plus VARIVAX). Here are a few things to know about ProQuad:

- It can be used as the first dose of MMR and VARIVAX.

- It can be used as the booster dose of MMR if your child also needs to have a chicken-pox injection.

- ProQuad can be given at the same time as the Hib and hepatitis B vaccines.

- You must wait at least one month between administration of the M-M-R II vaccine and ProQuad.

## Side Effects of the MMR Vaccine

The most common reactions associated with the MMR vaccine are soreness, redness, and swelling at the injection site, as well as a mild noncontagious rash, swelling of the lymph glands, mild to moderate fever, and temporary pain, stiffness, or swelling in the joints. In 5 to 15 percent of children, a fever higher than 103°F may occur, and it usually appears about seven to twelve days after the child receives the vaccine.

About 3 children out of 10,000 experience seizures related to a high fever (febrile seizure) after receiving MMR. This risk increases in children who receive MMRV. In very rare cases (less than 1 child out of 10,000), children experience coma, lowered consciousness, or a severe allergic reaction (e.g., swelling inside the mouth, breathing difficulties, low blood pressure).

One in every twenty-two thousand MMR vaccinations could cause a child to develop a temporary bleeding condition called idiopathic thrombocytopenic purpura, or ITP. This disorder is easily treated and is rarely dangerous. Studies indicate that children who had ITP and who later received the MMR vaccine did not have any recurrence of ITP.

## CONCERNS AND CONTROVERSIES

### MMR and Autism: Another Possibility

For more than a decade, there has been controversy about
the link between autism and the MMR vaccine announced
by Dr. Wakefield and published in *The Lancet* back in 1998.
I discussed that well-publicized debate in chapter 2 on safety
and vaccines. Even though the autism–MMR link was dis-
credited by the scientific community, there is more to the
MMR and autism story—beyond Wakefield—that most
people have not heard about, so I present it here.

Some researchers continue to suggest, if not somewhat
cautiously, that a connection between MMR and autism is
possible. One such individual, noted researcher Helen Ratajczak, explained her viewpoint in 2011 in the *Journal of Im-
munotoxicology*. In the article, Ratajczak, who has authored
and coauthored dozens of papers and is past president of the
Northeast Chapter of the Society of Toxicology, explains
the importance of the presence of human fetal DNA in the
M-M-R-II and VARIVAX (chicken-pox) vaccines.

She notes in her article that "documented causes of autism include genetic mutations and/or deletions, viral infections, and encephalitis following vaccination." Other facts
worth mentioning:

- The M-M-R II vaccine, which does not contain thi-
  merosol, was introduced in 1979 and was the only
  version of the vaccine available by 1983. Between
  1983 and 1990, autism in the United States rose
  dramatically, from 4 to 5 per 10,000 to 1 in 500.

- In 1988, two doses of M-M-R II were recommended
  for children who did not respond to the first injection. A dramatic increase of autism occurred along
  with the addition of the second dose of M-M-R II.

- Although the prevalence of autism per 10,000 increased by about 50 percent every two years between 1984 and 1990, during that same time span there were no changes in prevalence of mental retardation, traumatic brain injury, or speech/language impairment, "which suggests that the increase in autism is real."

Ratajczak further points out that the "MMR II vaccine is contaminated with human DNA from the cell line" and that "this human DNA could be the cause of the spikes in incidence." Another spike in the incidence of autism occurred in 1995 when the varicella (chicken-pox) vaccine was grown in human fetal tissue. She explains that "the incidence and prevalence data indicate the timing of introduction of vaccines and changes in the type and increasing number of vaccines given at one time implicate vaccines as a cause of autism."

To further support the possibility that vaccinations are associated with autism, Ratajczak points out that the immune system is especially sensitive in 2-month-old infants and that "a challenge by so many vaccines while the immune system is compromised might contribute to an onset of autism." In fact, she points to the possibility that "the vaccine organism itself could be a culprit." To illustrate this possibility, she mentions a hypothesis that suggests the pertussis toxin in the DPT vaccine "causes a separation of the G-alpha protein from retinoid receptors in genetically at-risk children." While this is a technical concept, like some others presented by Ratajczak, it provides a thought-provoking read concerning a possible link between autism and vaccinations. (Note 3 for this chapter provides a link to her paper.)

## Waning Immunity

In a 2011 study published in the *Canadian Medical Association Journal*, a research team analyzed a recent outbreak of mumps in Ontario, Canada (while similar outbreaks had occurred in New York and New Jersey), and announced that two doses of mumps vaccine are more effective than one. They emphasized the importance of making sure everyone, and especially older adolescents and young adults, be current on their mumps vaccinations.

Another observation from the study's authors was that while outbreaks of mumps in countries that have a two-dose vaccination policy (as do the United States and Canada) are fairly unusual, they have become more frequent since 2006. The authors suggested there may be some waning of immunity of people who receive two doses of vaccine. In that vein, the authors stated in the conclusion of their report: "Closely monitoring waning immunity will help to ensure that we have the necessary data for making policy decisions, such as whether a third dose of MMR vaccine is necessary or whether a different vaccine should be considered, and for evaluating the cost-effectiveness of the program." Whether the United States will eventually adopt a three-dose policy for MMR remains to be seen.

# CHAPTER 10

Chicken Pox (Varicella)

In the days before the introduction of a vaccine for chicken pox (varicella), some parents would send their children to chicken-pox parties. Here is how it worked: When a child got chicken pox, his or her parents would invite other children to come over and have a party so all the children would be exposed to the germ. All the kids would play together and share snacks. The idea was that the children could "get the chicken pox over with," which in turn reduced their chances of getting the disease later in life when it would be a much more serious problem. Chicken pox among children is typically (but not always) a mild, although uncomfortable, illness, but among adults there is a much greater chance of infection, pneumonia, encephalitis, and even death.

Today we have a vaccine for chicken pox. Although most parents choose the vaccine over the party—and such parties and playdates are still being held around the country—the varicella vaccine is the one parents are most likely to refuse for their children. One reason is that chicken pox is usually milder than other diseases for which there are vaccines, such as polio and pneumococcal meningitis. Another reason is that many parents realize that if they do not vaccinate their child he or she will benefit from the "herd immunity" provided by other children at the school. The theory of herd immunity proposes that when large numbers of a population are immune to a disease (e.g., they have been vaccinated) the chance that a susceptible individual (nonvaccinated) will have contact with an infectious person is small. In other words, it is a gamble, but one some parents are willing to take.

That being said, children who are not vaccinated for chicken pox can and do get the disease, and their cases can be mild, moderate, or severe. According to a study conducted by Kaiser Permanente Institute for Health Research in Colorado, children who do not get vaccinated for chicken pox are nine times more likely to get the disease than children who are vaccinated.

Perhaps your child has already received one or both varicella shots, or maybe you are unsure about the importance of this vaccine. In this chapter you will learn about chicken pox and the vaccine that was developed to help prevent this childhood disease.

## WHAT IS CHICKEN POX?

Chicken pox is a common illness that typically affects children, especially those younger than 12 years old. The disease is caused by the varicella-zoster virus (VZV), which results in a highly contagious infection characterized by an itchy rash all over the body.

Although the symptoms of chicken pox are generally mild, in rare cases the disease can be severe and even fatal (less than 1 out of every 10,000 cases). Chicken pox differs from most other childhood diseases managed with vaccines in that the virus can lie dormant in the body for decades and cause a different type of skin condition later in life called shingles. Children who get the varicella vaccine have a much greater chance of not getting chicken pox, but they may still develop shingles in their later years.

## Symptoms of Chicken Pox

The most prominent symptom of chicken pox is a red, itchy rash, but one or two days before it appears other symptoms may occur. These include fever, abdominal pain, headache, sore throat, and a general sick feeling. Once the rash begins, it usually first appears on the stomach or back and face before it spreads all over the body, including inside the mouth, nose, and ears. At first the rash looks like small red pimples, which then develop into blisters filled with clear fluid that turns cloudy. When the blisters break, they leave open sores that eventually crust over with scabs.

If your child has a skin condition such as eczema, the chicken-pox rash may be more severe. Generally, younger kids have milder symptoms and fewer blisters than older kids. Infants, children, and adolescents who have a weakened immune system usually experience a more severe form of chicken pox and are more likely to have complications. Those complications may include bacterial infections (in up to 5 percent of cases), pneumonia (23 out of every 10,000 cases), brain inflammation (encephalitis; 1 in every 10,000 cases), decreased platelets, arthritis, and hepatitis. Generally, anyone who scratches the rash and breaks the blisters risks developing a skin infection. Chicken pox is also an important risk factor for a severe streptococcal disease (group A) often referred to as "flesh-eating disease," which is very rare.

Up to 20 percent of children who either develop chicken pox or get the vaccine will develop shingles later in life. That's because the VZV can remain inactive in the spinal cord and become active in later life, causing itching, pain, and rash.

## How Chicken Pox Is Transmitted

Chicken pox can be transmitted through direct contact with someone who is infected with the virus (even if he or she does not display any symptoms yet) or through the air when an infected person sneezes, coughs, or laughs. Less often, the disease can be spread when someone has direct contact with a person who has an active shingles infection.

A person who has the varicella virus is contagious one to two days before the rash appears until all the blisters have formed scabs. If your child gets chicken pox, he or she will need to stay out of school until all the blisters have dried, which usually takes one week. It usually takes ten to twenty-one days after contact with an infected person for someone to develop chicken pox.

Most kids who have a brother or sister who has chicken pox will get the disease as well if they have not already had the disease or the vaccine. If you have a child with chicken pox, keep him or her away from any unvaccinated siblings as much as possible.

## Risk Factors for Chicken Pox

Factors that will increase a child's risk of contracting chicken pox if he or she is not immune include:

- Direct contact with someone who is infected

- Sharing personal items such as eating utensils or drinking containers with someone who has chicken pox

- Having a compromised immune system because of cancer, chemotherapy, HIV/AIDS, use of immuno-suppressant drugs, or presence of a severe illness

- Being a newborn whose mother never contracted chicken pox before pregnancy

- Traveling abroad, because chicken pox is much more common outside the United States (also see chapter 16, "Vaccines for Young Travelers")

## Treatment of Chicken Pox

Because chicken pox is caused by a virus, your doctor will not prescribe antibiotics. However, if your child develops a skin infection from scratching the sores, an antibiotic may be ordered to treat the infection. The antiviral medication acyclovir can be prescribed for some people who get chicken pox and who are at risk for complications. Acyclovir must be taken within twenty-four hours after the rash appears to be effective. Because acyclovir can cause significant side effects, it should only be used when necessary.

Typically, treatment of chicken pox involves relieving the discomfort caused by the rash. Wet, cool compresses or baths in cool water (with oatmeal bath products) every three to four hours can help relieve the itch. Calamine lotion can be applied to the rash but not on the face. If your child has chicken pox in the mouth, avoid foods that are acidic or salty. Acetaminophen can help relieve pain if your child has mouth blisters.

To help children not scratch the rash, put socks or mittens on their hands, especially at night. Keep their fingernails trimmed and clean to help prevent breaking of blisters and infection.

In most cases, chicken-pox infections are fairly mild. However, if any of the following symptoms occur, contact your physician: fever that lasts for more than four days or is greater than 102°F, severe cough or difficulty breathing, sensitivity to light, difficulty walking, confusion, vomiting, or stiff neck.

## Chicken Pox During Pregnancy

Women who contract chicken pox during early pregnancy can transmit the virus to the fetus. Therefore, any pregnant woman who has never had chicken pox but has been exposed to the disease, especially in the first twenty weeks of pregnancy, should contact her doctor immediately.

Exposing the fetus to chicken pox during pregnancy can

result in a variety of complications. In about 2 percent of cases, the infant can develop limb deformities, eye damage, brain atrophy, mental retardation, scarring of the skin, and low birth weight. Varicella virus can cause spontaneous abortion or death of the infant soon after birth.

If you are pregnant and already had chicken pox in the past, you will pass along immunity to your child, who will be protected from the infection for the first few months of life.

## ABOUT THE VARICELLA VACCINE

A varicella vaccine was developed in Japan in the 1970s and licensed for use in 1988 in both Japan and Korea. The United States started routine immunization with a varicella vaccine in 1995, and ten years later a combination vaccine (MMR plus varicella, called ProQuad) was licensed for use.

Before the varicella vaccine was introduced in the United States, 3 to 4 million cases of chicken pox occurred each year and approximately one hundred deaths were associated with the disease per year. Since immunization for chicken pox started, the number and severity of cases have declined dramatically. At first, only one injection was recommended by the CDC. However, because of continued outbreaks of the disease, the CDC recommended a second dose of varicella vaccine for all children starting in 2006. While this second dose appears to have reduced the incidence of chicken pox, outbreaks still continue with some regularity every year, resulting in hundreds of cases across the country.

The current varicella vaccine is about 70 to 85 percent effective at preventing a mild infection and more than 95 percent effective at preventing a moderate to severe case of the disease. If a vaccinated child does get chicken pox, it is usually a very mild case with mild or no fever, fewer skin lesions, and recovery within a few days.

## VARIVAX

VARIVAX (Merck) is the only varicella vaccine licensed in the United States. Each 0.5 mL dose contains about 25 mg of sucrose, 12.5 mg of hydrolyzed gelatin, 3.2 mg of sodium chloride, 0.5 mg of monosodium glutamate, 0.45 mg of sodium phosphate dibasic, 0.08 mg of potassium phosphate monobasic, 0.08 mg of potassium chloride, trace quantities of sodium phosphate monobasic, EDTA, neomycin, and fetal bovine serum. VARIVAX does not contain preservatives.

## ProQuad

The ProQuad vaccine is a combination of MMR plus varicella. A full explanation of this vaccine is in chapter 9 on MMR.

## Who Should Get the Varicella Vaccine

Experts recommend the varicella vaccine for the following individuals:

- All children aged 12 to 18 months.

- All older children and adults who have never had chicken pox, who have never been vaccinated, or who have had only one dose of the vaccine.

- Anyone who has never had chicken pox or the vaccine and who is exposed to the disease should get the vaccine within seventy-two hours to probably prevent or significantly reduce the severity of the disease.

Healthy kids who have had chicken pox do not need to get the vaccine, because they will likely have lifelong protection against the illness. All fifty states plus the District of Columbia require varicella immunization (or proof of immunity) for children before they enter school. See the

Immunization Action Coalition entry in the appendices for links to specific information for each state.

## The Varicella Schedule

The CDC recommends the following vaccination schedule for the varicella vaccine:

- First dose at age 12 to 15 months

- Booster dose at 4 to 6 years

The second dose may be given before age 4 years if at least three months have passed since your child received the first dose. For children ages 12 months through 12 years, a minimum of three months should pass between doses. However, if the second dose is administered at least four weeks after the first dose, it is considered valid.

The catch-up schedule for varicella vaccination is as follows:

- For children ages 7 to 18 years who have no evidence of immunity, they should get two doses if not previously vaccinated or the second dose if they received the first dose.

- For children ages 7 to 12 years, the minimum interval between doses is three months. However, if the second dose was given at least twenty-eight days after the first dose it is considered to be valid.

- For children ages 13 years and older, the minimum interval between doses is twenty-eight days.

## When to Delay or Avoid the Varicella Vaccine

Some children should delay getting the chicken-pox vaccine or avoid it altogether. Here are examples:

- Your child should not get the vaccine if he or she has ever had a life-threatening allergic reaction to a previous dose of varicella vaccine or to gelatin or to the antibiotic neomycin.

- Delay the vaccine if your child is moderately or severely ill at the time the shot is scheduled.

- Consult your doctor if your child has HIV/AIDS or any other disease that affects the immune system, is being treated with drugs that impact the immune system (e.g., steroids), has cancer, is receiving cancer treatment, or has recently received a transfusion or received other blood products.

- Pregnant women should not receive the vaccine until after they have delivered their child.

In addition, women who plan to get pregnant and who need the vaccine should receive it at least one month before they get pregnant

## Side Effects of the Varicella Vaccination

Most children who get the vaccine for chicken pox experience mild or no symptoms. Reactions are usually more likely to occur after the first dose than after the second. The most common side effects are soreness and/or swelling at the injection site, which occurs in about 20 percent of children and up to one-third of adolescents. Fever develops in up to 10 percent of children, and a mild rash, which can appear up to one month after the vaccination, occurs in about 4 percent. Although it is possible for these individuals to infect other members of the household, it rarely happens. In rare cases, seizures caused by fever, pneumonia, and low blood count have been reported after chicken-pox vaccination.

In children who get the combination vaccine ProQuad (MMR plus varicella), rash and fever are reported more often than when they get the vaccines individually. Specifically, fever within forty-two days of being vaccinated occurs in about 22 out of every 100 children vaccinated compared with about 15 percent in children who receive two separate shots. Children who receive the MMRV vaccine are also more likely to experience febrile seizures (about 8 out of every 10,000 children vaccinated) during the five to twelve days after vaccination than the 4 out of every 10,000 children who receive two separate shots.

## CONCERNS AND CONTROVERSIES

One concern parents have about the varicella vaccine is that it is scheduled to be given at the same time—between 12 and 15 months of age—as the combination vaccine MMR. The worry is that injecting four viruses plus all the vaccine additives into such a young child increases the risk of side effects and possibly long-term complications. The CDC assures parents that the risk of side effects from getting both vaccines at the same time—or getting the combination vaccine containing both MMR and varicella—exposes children to minimal risks. Here is a summary of the CDC's stance:

Whether your child receives one or two shots, the amount of protection against the diseases is the same. Both shots can be given at the same doctor's visit. Although one shot may be less traumatic for the child than two, worries about the ingredients in the vaccines remain. As mentioned previously, however, administration of the MMRV vaccine is associated with a greater risk of side effects.

# CHAPTER 11

Polio

On May 19, 2011, Secretary of Health and Human Services Kathleen Sebelius spoke at the World Health Assembly, saying there were "two major issues for the U.S.: the eradication of polio, as concerns remain in countries where the disease is endemic, such as Afghanistan, India, Nigeria, and Pakistan, with outbreaks in other nations, and maintaining the stocks of smallpox virus, which has already been eradicated."

Thanks to initiation of polio vaccinations in the mid-1950s in the United States, cases of polio occurring through natural infection (as compared with cases developing from the vaccine, which is discussed in this chapter) were eliminated from the United States by 1979 and from the Western Hemisphere by 1991. Before that time, however, nearly sixty thousand cases of the devastating disease were reported at the height of the polio epidemic in 1952, with more than three thousand deaths in the United States.

Six countries in the world—Afghanistan, Egypt, India, Niger, Nigeria, and Pakistan—still have polio circulating in the population, which means the virus could infiltrate other countries. Therefore, until polio has been eliminated around the world it is important to continue vaccinating children against polio in the United States. Thus, this chapter explores the disease known as polio and the vaccine used to prevent it.

## WHAT IS POLIO?

Polio, also known as poliomyelitis, is a contagious viral disease that has been a serious problem since ancient times. The disease affects the nervous system and, in rare cases, causes paralysis. Polio most commonly affects young children.

Although it is rare to see cases of polio today in the United States, there was a time this was not so. During the late 1940s and early 1950s, an average of more than thirty-five thousand cases per year were reported in the United States. Once the Salk inactivated poliovirus vaccine (IPV) was introduced in 1955 the number of cases dropped dramatically to less than twenty-five hundred in 1957. By 1961, only sixty-one cases of paralytic polio (the most serious type of polio; see "Symptoms of Polio") were reported.

The last time anyone developed a case of naturally occurring paralytic polio in the United States was in 1979, when an outbreak occurred among the Amish. "Naturally occurring polio," or "wild poliovirus," refers to instances of the disease that develop from the virus that is found naturally in the environment. This contrasts with vaccine-associated paralytic polio, which is caused by the live oral poliovirus vaccine (OPV). This vaccine, as you will learn later in this chapter, is no longer used in the United States.

However, before the OPV was withdrawn from the U.S. market in 2000 scores of cases of vaccine-associated paralytic polio (the worst type; see "Symptoms of Polio") developed in the United States. From 1980 through 1999, there were 162 confirmed cases of paralytic polio. Eight of the individuals got the disease outside the United States and came home with it. The remaining 154 cases were caused by OPV.

There is yet another type of polio called vaccine-derived

poliovirus (VDPV), which is a strain of poliovirus that was initially in the OPV but has since mutated and now acts more like naturally occurring virus. This makes VDPV more easily transmitted to people who are not vaccinated against polio and who make contact with the virus. Fortunately, VDPV is extremely rare.

In 2005, an unvaccinated, immunocompromised infant living in Minnesota had VDPV in stool. Authorities believed the child caught the virus from someone who had received the live oral vaccine in another country several months earlier. An additional seven unvaccinated children in the original child's community also were found to have poliovirus infection, but none of them developed paralysis.

## Symptoms of Polio

In about 95 percent of cases of polio, individuals do not experience symptoms. This type of the disease is called asymptomatic polio. In 4 to 8 percent of cases, the disease causes symptoms and can appear in three different forms:

- *Abortive polio,* a mild form characterized by flu-like symptoms such as diarrhea, fever, sore throat, feeling unwell, and a mild upper respiratory infection. Anyone who gets this form of the disease usually makes a full recovery.

- *Nonparalytic polio,* which is associated with aseptic meningitis and symptoms such as a stiff neck and sensitivity to light. Full recovery can be expected.

- *Paralytic polio,* a severe, debilitating form of the disease that occurs in 0.1 to 2 percent of cases. In this form, the virus enters the bloodstream and attacks the nerves. In some cases, it affects the respiratory system and causes paralysis of the arms and legs. It can even cause death.

Even though the acute illness usually lasts less than two weeks, any damage to the nervous system can last a lifetime. In the past, some people who got polio never regained complete use of their arms or legs, while others developed post-polio syndrome thirty or more years after the first illness. Post-polio syndrome speeds up normal weakness associated with aging. Today, people classified as "baby boomers" are those typically affected by post-polio syndrome.

## How Polio Is Transmitted

Polio is transmitted mainly by ingesting materials that have been contaminated with the virus, which is found in stool. Common ways to spread the virus are drinking contaminated water and not washing hands thoroughly after using the bathroom.

## Risk Factors for Polio

Although polio is rare in the United States, it has not been eliminated entirely. Therefore, risk factors for the disease should still be heeded. They include:

- Not getting vaccinated or not completing vaccination for the disease

- Traveling to countries where polio is still a problem (areas of Asia and Africa)

- Recent or previous removal of the tonsils (tonsillectomy), which exposes nerve endings to the virus

- Immunodeficiency, such as presence of HIV/AIDS

## ABOUT THE POLIO VACCINE

In 1952, Dr. Jonas Salk developed the IPV, also called the Salk vaccine, which was designed for subcutaneous injection. The IPV contains strains of the three strains of polioviruses (types 1, 2, and 3), and the original vaccine was grown in monkey kidney cell culture.

The Salk vaccine was put to the test in clinical trials in 1954, and once researchers saw a dramatic drop in the number of polio cases the U.S. government granted approval for distribution in 1955. This same formulation was used until 1987, when a more potent version of inactivated poliovirus vaccine was introduced. This vaccine, which is prepared using human cell culture, is the one still used today.

The other type of polio vaccine, developed in 1958 by Dr. Albert Sabin, is the OPV. This is a live vaccine, which means it contains live attenuated (weakened) strains of the three polioviruses. In 2000, the Advisory Committee on Immunization Practices recommended discontinuing use of the OPV to eliminate the risk of vaccine-associated paralytic poliomyelitis. The OPV is still used in many other parts of the world.

### Ipol

Ipol is the only polio vaccine currently used in the United States. This inactivated vaccine, produced by Sanofi Pasteur SA, contains three strains of poliovirus grown in monkey kidney cells. In addition to the strains, each 0.5 mL dose contains 0.5 percent of 2-phenoxyethanol and no more than 0.02 percent of formaldehyde as preservatives, as well as less than 5ng of neomycin, 200 ng of streptomycin, and 25 ng of polymyxin B, which are used during production. Residual calf serum protein is less than 1 ppm.

## Pediarix

This vaccine is a combination of DTaP, hepatitis B, and polio. Details about Pediarix can be found in chapter 5 on DTP.

## Kinrix

The Kinrix vaccine is a combination of DTaP and polio. Details about the vaccine can be found in chapter 5 on DTP.

## Who Should Get the Polio Vaccine

Any child age 2 months and older should be immunized against polio. If you and your children are planning to travel outside the United States, especially to Africa and Asia, where polio is still a problem, make sure all of you have received all the polio vaccinations.

All fifty states plus the District of Columbia require immunization against polio before children can enter school. See the Immunization Action Coalition entry in the appendices for links to specific information for each state.

## The Polio Schedule

The current vaccination schedule for polio consists of four doses of IPV and is as follows:

- First dose at 2 months

- Second dose at 4 months

- Third dose at age 6 to 18 months

- The fourth and booster dose at age 4 to 6 years

Children who receive three doses of the IPV vaccine before age 4 should receive a fourth dose before or when they begin school. Children do not need to get the fourth dose if they were given the third dose after age 4.

## When to Delay or Avoid the Polio Vaccine

In some cases, your child should delay or avoid the polio vaccine. For example:

- If your child has a moderate or severe illness when he or she is scheduled to get the vaccine, you should wait until the illness passes.

- Your child should avoid the vaccine if he or she has ever had a life-threatening allergic reaction to neomycin, streptomycin, or polymyxin.

- Your child should not get the vaccine if he or she has ever had a severe allergic reaction to a polio shot.

- Your child should not get the vaccine if he or she has received cancer chemotherapy or radiation treatment within the past three months.

- Tell your doctor before your child gets the polio vaccine if he or she has a bleeding or blood-clotting disorder, a history of seizures, or a weak immune system or bruises easily,

## Side Effects of the Polio Vaccine

Most children who get the polio vaccine experience mild or no symptoms. Reactions are usually more likely to occur after the first dose than after the rest of the series. The most common side effect is irritability, which occurs in up to 60 percent or more of children within a few hours of receiving the injection. Other common and less serious side effects include redness, pain, swelling, and a lump where the injection is given; low fever, joint pain, body aches, drowsiness, and vomiting. In rare cases, there is fainting, seizures, or high fever (that occurs within a few hours or a few days after the injection).

## CONCERNS AND CONTROVERSIES

The primary concerns about polio are (1) eliminating it in the countries where it still circulates, which are Afghanistan, Egypt, India, Niger, Nigeria, and Pakistan; and (2) ensuring the virus does not get imported into a country where an insufficient number of people are immunized, which could result in it spreading among the population; with the ultimate goal of (3) eliminating polio entirely from the planet. One other concern is that many countries still use the OPV, which carries a very small but potent risk of actually causing paralytic polio.

# CHAPTER 12

Hepatitis A

Hepatitis A is a disease you may not hear about very often, and there is a good reason: in the United States, the incidence of new cases declined by 92 percent from 1995 to 2007, from 12 cases per 100,000 people to 1 per 100,000 people. Some other good news is that the greatest declines in hepatitis A have been among children and in states where routine vaccination of children against the disease has been recommended since 1999.

But the fight is not over yet. The less-than-good news is that hepatitis A is still a significant health problem. Hepatitis A infection continues to be one of the most frequently reported diseases that are preventable with a vaccine, even though the vaccine was introduced in the United States in 1995. One reason hepatitis A continues to be a problem is that children are the ones most likely to become infected and, because they usually don't experience any symptoms, they can unknowingly spread it to others. Hepatitis A is especially a concern among children living in underdeveloped and developing countries.

The goal in this chapter is to enhance your knowledge of hepatitis A and the vaccines that were developed to prevent it.

## WHAT IS HEPATITIS A?

Hepatitis A is a type of liver disease caused by the hepatitis A virus (HAV.). The virus can cause the liver to become inflamed, but fortunately, it rarely causes lasting damage. However, the hepatitis A virus is very resilient—it is able to withstand the body's highly acidic digestive tract and live for more than a week at room temperature on surfaces. The virus can survive up to ten months in water, which is why it can be found in shellfish living in water contaminated by sewage.

### Symptoms of Hepatitis A

If your child has been exposed to HAV, it can take from two to seven weeks before any signs of the disease appear. If symptoms do occur—and many children do not experience symptoms—they can include:

- Clay-colored stools

- Dark urine

- Fatigue

- Itching

- Jaundice

- Loss of appetite

- Low-grade fever

- Nausea and vomiting

- Pain on the right side under the rib cage

Because all types of hepatitis (hepatitis A, B, and C) cause similar symptoms, your child will need a blood test to determine if he or she has hepatitis A or another form of the disease.

When symptoms do appear, they are typically mild but may last for up to several months. The majority of people with hepatitis A recover within three months.

## How Hepatitis A Is Transmitted

Hepatitis A virus is found in the stools of infected individuals, and it is spread mainly when someone eats food or drinks water that has been contaminated with the organisms from the infected feces. Therefore, anyone who has contact with an infected person's stool—for example, changing a diaper or not washing hands after using the bathroom—can spread the virus. An infected individual who works in a restaurant and who does not wash his or her hands after using the bathroom could spread the virus to fellow employees and to people who eat food touched by the infected worker.

Hepatitis A virus can also lurk in high concentrations in some shellfish, such as raw oysters or undercooked clams or mussels. If you and your children are in a country where hepatitis A is common, untreated tap water, uncooked foods, and foods washed in water contaminated by fecal matter could carry the virus. You cannot get hepatitis A through kissing or sharing utensils.

According to the Centers for Disease Control and Prevention, about 9 percent of reported cases of hepatitis A occur among children or employees in day-care centers. Another 13 percent of reported cases in the United States are associated with international travel, most often in Mexico, Central America, or South America.

Infected people are most likely to spread the virus one week before and up to one week after the appearance of symptoms or elevation of liver enzymes, which is one way doctors can detect the disease. Therefore, people can easily spread the disease and not even know they are doing so. Infected infants and children can spread the virus in their stool for longer periods of time than can adults, up to several months. Therefore, children play a big role in transmitting HAV. In fact, about half of all cases of people with hepatitis A had household contact with young children who had been infected with the virus.

## Risk Factors for Hepatitis A

For children, the most important risk factor for contracting hepatitis A is international travel (especially to South or Central America or Asia). For adults, risk factors also include living in a nursing home or rehabilitation facility, working in health care or in the food or sewage industry, and intravenous drug use.

## Treatment of Hepatitis A

Hepatitis A is a condition for which there are no specific treatments. If your child contracts a severe case of hepatitis A, rest is recommended, and avoiding fatty foods may help ward off vomiting. If you know your child has been exposed to HAV, your doctor may recommend he or she get immune globulin (immunoglobulin; GamaSTAn, Gammar-P) for maximum protection, if exposure to the virus was within two weeks. Immune globulin is a drug that contains antibodies that destroy the hepatitis A virus and provides protection but only for three to five months. (Also see chapter 16, "Vaccines for young travelers.")

## ABOUT THE HEPATITIS A VACCINES

As of 2011, there were two hepatitis A vaccines available, plus a third vaccine designed to prevent both hepatitis A and B. Hepatitis A vaccines are for people age 12 months and older, and the primary dose should be given at least two weeks before any expected exposure to hepatitis A virus. Once your child receives the first dose, it begins to provide protection within four weeks. The booster dose is necessary for long-term protection. Hepatitis A vaccine is usually 100 percent effective if both doses are administered before exposure to the virus.

## Havrix

Havrix (GlaxoSmithKline; approved 1995) contains inactivated virus adsorbed on aluminum hydroxide. Ingredients present in each 0.5 mL dose of Havrix include amino acid supplement (0.3 percent weight/volume), phosphate-buffered saline solution, polysorbate 20 (0.05 mg/mL), no more than 0.1 mg/mL formalin, and no more than 40 ng/mL neomycin sulfate. Havrix does not contain preservatives, but if your child is allergic to latex take note. Havrix is available in vials and two types of prefilled syringes. One type of syringe has a tip cap that may contain latex, and the other has a tip cap and rubber plunger that contains latex. The vial stopper does not contain latex.

## Vaqta

Vaqta (Merck & Company; approved 1996) is a vaccine designed for intramuscular injection and contains inactivated virus absorbed onto about 0.225 mg of aluminum hydroxyphosphate sulfate. Each 0.5 mL dose consists of a minute amount of bovine albumin, less than 0.8 mcg of formaldehyde, 35 mcg of sodium borate, 0.9 percent sodium chloride, and less than 10 ppb of neomycin. There are no preservatives in Vaqta.

## Twinrix

Twinrix (GlaxoSmithKline) is a bivalent vaccine, which means it was designed to help prevent two conditions, hepatitis A and hepatitis B. The vaccine contains components from Havrix and Engerix-B (hepatitis B vaccine, see chapter 3) and is administered via intramuscular injection. Each 1.0 mL dose of Twinrix contains about 0.45 mg of aluminum as aluminum phosphate and aluminum hydroxide, amino acids, sodium chloride, phosphate buffer, polysorbate 20, no more than 0.1 mg of formalin, no more than 5 percent yeast protein, and no more than 20 ng of neomycin. Twinrix is available in vials and prefilled syringes. One type of syringe has a tip cap that may contain latex, and the other has a tip cap and rubber plunger that contains latex. The vial stopper does not contain latex. No preservatives are present in Twinrix.

Children can receive their booster dose of Vaqta at six to twelve months after receiving their primary dose of another inactivated hepatitis A vaccine (Havrix).

## Who Should Get the Hepatitis A Vaccine

The hepatitis A vaccine is recommended for the following individuals:

- All children ages 12 through 23 months

- Anyone age 1 year or older who is traveling to a country that has a high or intermediate prevalence of hepatitis A, such as those in Central or South America, Mexico, Asia, Africa, and eastern Europe

- Children and adolescents up to age 18 years who live in communities or states where routine vaccination has been implemented because there is a high incidence of the disease

- Anyone who has chronic liver disease

- People who use street drugs

Seventeen states require that children be vaccinated against hepatitis A before they enter school. See the Immunization

Action Coalition entry in the appendices for links to specific information for each state.

## The Hepatitis A Schedule

The CDC recommends the following schedule for the hepatitis A vaccine:

- Administer two doses between the ages of 12 and 23 months.

- The second dose should be given at least 6 months after the first dose.

- The vaccine is also recommended for children older than 23 months who are at high risk for the disease; that is, those who live in areas where vaccination programs target older children, when children are at increased risk for the disease (e.g., during foreign travel), or when immunity against the disease is desired.

The CDC's catch-up schedule for hepatitis A can be seen in the appendices.

## When to Delay or Avoid the Hepatitis A Vaccine

Not everyone is a candidate for the hepatitis A vaccine. Your child should delay receiving the injection or avoid it altogether based on the following factors:

- Delay the injection if your child has a moderate or severe illness at the time the shot is scheduled. You should consult your physician.

- Avoid the injection if your child had a life-threatening allergic reaction to a previous dose of hepatitis A vaccine.

- Avoid the injection if your child has a severe allergy to any component in the vaccine. (See description of vaccines in this chapter.)

## Side Effects of the Hepatitis A Vaccine

Most children who get the hepatitis A vaccine experience
mild or no side effects. The most common response is soreness where the injection is given. Studies involving Havrix
show, for example, that 21 percent of children experience
injection-site soreness, while it reportedly affects up to 42
percent of children ages 12 through 23 months who get Vaqta.
Headache has been reported in less than 9 percent of children
who get Havrix, and between 1 and 10 percent experience
nausea, loss of appetite, fatigue, fever, redness and swelling at
the injection site, and malaise. Injection-site pain (18.7 percent) and headache (2.3 percent) have been noted in children
ages 2 through 18 years who receive Vaqta. These side effects
typically last one or two days.

On rare occasions, a serious allergic reaction occurs
within a few minutes to a few hours after receiving a hepatitis A shot.

## CONCERNS AND CONTROVERSIES

If there is one childhood vaccine that does not stir up much
controversy, it would likely be the one for hepatitis A. It has
not been the subject of recalls, unusual complications, or
similar concerns. Some parents argue, however, that since
the disease is typically very mild and one that does not often
affect children perhaps there is no need for a vaccine. However, hepatitis A can cause community-wide outbreaks, be
expensive to treat, and be a burden on a community's health
resources.

One concern about hepatitis A was recently highlighted
in the results of a study published in *Pediatrics*. Researchers
looked at the number of cases of hepatitis A in Minnesota

from 2007 through 2009 associated with international adoptees. During that time period, ten cases of hepatitis A related to contact with an infected adoptee. A total of twenty-one recently arrived foreign-born adoptees, all younger than 5 years, were identified during the study period, and only six of the children had symptoms.

The take-home message from this study is that doctors, adopting parents, and others who will have close contact with the adoptees should be aware that young children recently adopted from areas where hepatitis A is endemic may have the disease and that many of them may be asymptomatic. New adoptees should be screened for hepatitis A and parents and other close contacts should be informed about preventive measures, including vaccination.

# CHAPTER 13

Meningococcal Disease

In mid-April 2011, officials with the Los Angeles County Department of Public Health announced that a bacterial illness that could cause meningitis was on the rise. The illness was meningococcal disease, a name that does not roll off the tongue as easily as do measles, chicken pox, and the flu, yet it can be even more deadly and life altering than these other diseases. The officials were concerned because seven cases of meningococcal disease had been reported since mid-March and a total of twenty-one had been reported for the entire year in 2010.

Meningococcal disease attacks the blood and the meninges, which is the thin lining covering the spinal cord and brain. If this explanation sounds familiar, that's because I have already discussed another type of serious bacterial disease that can affect the blood and meninges—pneumococcal disease. However, the main difference between these two types of bacterial diseases is in the microorganisms responsible. Even though the causative germs are different, they can still be deadly. And they both can be prevented with vaccination. In this chapter I explore meningococcal disease and the vaccines designed to prevent it.

## WHAT IS MENINGOCOCCAL DISEASE?

Meningococcal disease includes meningococcal meningitis and meningococcemia, both of which are caused by the bacterium *Neisseria meningitidis*. A person may have either meningococcal meningitis or meningococcemia or both at the same time.

The culprit responsible for meningococcal disease can rapidly race through the body and result in death if there is not enough time for the body's immune system to mount an effective defense once the disease has taken hold. Such a failure by the immune system can happen if an individual has not been immunized. Therefore, even if meningococcal disease is recognized early and appropriate treatment is administered, the disease may progress rapidly and cause death within twenty-four to forty-eight hours after symptoms begin.

For far too many people, the disease takes its toll. Meningococcal disease affects more than five hundred thousand people each year, resulting in more than fifty thousand deaths around the world. Up to 1 in 7 people who contract meningococcal disease die from it, and about 20 percent of those who survive the disease experience permanent and life-altering side effects, including amputation, seizures, paralysis, learning disabilities, and hearing loss.

People of any age can get meningococcal disease, but it is most common in children younger than 5 years of age. Compared with other persons their age, college freshman, especially if they live in a dormitory environment, are at a slightly increased risk for developing meningococcal disease.

Five serogroups are responsible for the majority of meningococcal disease around the world: A, B, C, Y, and W-135. These serogroups are distributed disproportionately and vary from geographic region to region and even change over time. Although it is not possible to identify exactly which serogroups will cause most cases of disease from year to year, the three that have been most prominent in the United

States in recent years are serogroups B, C, and Y. The vaccines that have been developed to prevent meningococcal disease have been formulated to prevent four of the five serogroups (excluding B).

## SYMPTOMS OF MENINGOCOCCAL DISEASE

Symptoms of meningococcal disease can develop rapidly, sometimes in a matter of a few hours after exposure, and can vary widely. They can be difficult to detect in infants at first, because they mimic symptoms of other conditions and include lethargy, irritability, vomiting, and poor feeding. As the diseases progresses, patients of any age may experience seizures. Other common signs and symptoms include:

- Sudden high fever

- Severe, persistent headache

- Stiff neck

- High-pitched or moaning cry (infants)

- Jerky or stiff movements or floppiness (infants and toddlers)

- Bulging or tense soft spot (infants)

- High sensitivity to bright lights

- Drowsiness

- Joint pain

- Confusion or other mental changes

- Rapid breathing

A purple or reddish rash may be a sign of blood poisoning. If you press a glass against the rash and the skin does not turn white, seek immediate medical attention.

Antibiotics are the normal treatment for meningococcal disease, but despite immediate care, 10 to 15 percent of patients die. Among those who survive, complications such as permanent brain damage, hearing loss, kidney failure, loss of limbs, or chronic nervous system damage can occur.

## HOW MENINGOCOCCAL DISEASE IS TRANSMITTED

*N. meningitidis* bacteria are most often found in the nose and throat, and so meningococcal disease is spread by direct contact with the microorganisms in respiratory or oral secretions (e.g., sputum, nasal mucus, and saliva) through coughing, sneezing, kissing, and other intimate contact. Symptoms can appear as quickly as a few hours after exposure, but the usual incubation period is three to four days, ranging up to ten.

### Risk Factors for Meningococcal Disease

It is estimated that up to 10 percent of the population is carrying *N. meningitidis* bacteria in their throat and nose at any given time. However, most people exposed to *N. meningitidis* don't get sick. Experts are not certain why only a few people develop invasive meningococcal disease, but it is likely a combination of factors, including genetics, the state of their immune system, environmental factors (e.g., overcrowding, exposure to smoke), and/or physical factors that increase one's risk for developing disease.

Some of the risk factors for contracting meningococcal disease are associated with the way the disease is transmitted. A few studies have pointed out several interesting ways the disease has been shown to spread, especially among youngsters and adolescents, so parents, take note.

For example, a study from Johns Hopkins Bloomberg

School of Public Health showed that among young people in grades 9 through 12 marijuana use (i.e., sharing joints), nightclub attendance, and upper respiratory infections symptoms were shown to be risk factors. Another study, conducted at the University of London, evaluated 15- to 19-year-olds who had meningococcal disease. When the researchers analyzed each case, they found that intimate kissing with many partners, being a university student, and having been born prematurely were risk factors for the disease.

## Treatment of Meningococcal Disease

Early treatment is important because it can improve outcome and decrease the risk of complications. Antibiotics are the first course of treatment, including penicillin G, cefotaxime, ceftriaxone, rifampin, or ciprofloxacin. Corticosteroids can be prescribed to reduce the risk of complications, such as hearing loss.

# ABOUT THE MENINGOCOCCAL VACCINES

Currently there are three FDA-approved vaccines to help prevent meningococcal disease: Menomune, a polysaccharide vaccine that has been available in the United States since the 1970s; Menactra, a conjugate vaccine that was first approved in 2005; and Menveo, another conjugate vaccine. These vaccines are 85 to 100 percent effective in preventing the four kinds of the meningococcus germ (types A, C, Y, and W-135) that are responsible for about 70 percent of cases of meningococcal disease in the United States. Type B is another meningococcus germ, and it accounts for about one-third of meningococcal disease in adolescents, but none of the current vaccines include protection against this microorganism.

Here is more information you should know about each of the meningococcal vaccines. I use the acronym for both of the two basic types of vaccine:

- *MCV4*, which is meningococcal conjugated vaccine with four serogroups; and

- *MPSV4*, which is meningococcal polysaccharide vaccine with the four serogroups

## Menomune

The Menomune vaccine was the first meningococcal vaccine licensed in the United States and is approved for individuals ages 2 and older. Menomune is an MPSV4 prepared with antigens from *N. meningitidis* groups A, C, Y, and W-135. In addition to the four antigens, each 0.5 mL dose contains 2.5 to 5.0 mg of lactose added as a stabilizer. Vaccine from a multidose vial also contains thimerosal, providing 25 mcg of mercury.

## Menactra

The Menactra vaccine (Sanofi Pasteur) is an MCV4 approved for use in individuals ages 9 months to 55 years. Menactra was originally approved by the FDA in January 2005 for people ages 11 to 55 years. In October 2007, the FDA lowered the minimum age to 2 years. Then in April 2011, yet another change was made as the FDA extended use of the vaccine to include infants and toddlers as young as 9 months of age. As of mid-2011, Menactra was the only meningococcal vaccine licensed for use in children as young as 9 months old.

In October 2010, the ACIP voted to add a recommendation for a booster shot of the vaccine for adolescents at age 16 if they had first received the vaccine at age 11 or 12. The recommendations became official in January 2011, after the ACIP determined from studies that protection from the vaccine fades within five years.

Menactra contains the four *N. meningitidis* serogroup polysaccharide antigens, and the production process involves the use of formaldehyde, ammonium sulfate, sodium phosphate, and sodium chloride. Each 0.5 mL dose of the vaccine contains each of the meningococcal polysaccharides as well as no more than 2.66 mcg of formaldehyde.

## Menveo

The Menveo vaccine (Novartis) is approved for use in individuals ages 2 to 55 years. It is an MCV4 vaccine containing *N. meningitidis* serogroups A, C, Y, and W-135 oligosaccharides (a type of polysaccharide). The production process involves use of a culture containing yeast and amino acids. Each dose of the vaccine contains the four serotypes and no more than 0.30 mcg of formaldehyde. The vials and stoppers for administering the vaccine do not contain latex.

## Who Should Get the Meningococcal Disease Vaccine

Although the meningococcal vaccine is now available for children as young as 9 months old, the vast majority of children do not need to be vaccinated until they are older. (See "The Meningococcal Disease Schedules.") The CDC recommends the vaccine for all adolescents as they enter middle school (ages 11 to 12 years) and high school (15 years old) and for all first-year college students who live in dormitories or similar close quarters. The vaccine is also recommended for anyone who has had their spleen removed, people who work in certain laboratories, and individuals who travel to areas where meningococcal disease is endemic.

Twenty states require that children be vaccinated against meningococcal disease before they enter school. See the Immunization Action Coalition entry in the appendices for links to specific information for each state.

## The Meningococcal Disease Schedule

The CDC recommends the following vaccination schedule for meningococcal vaccines for children:

- Administer MCV4 to children at ages 11 through 12 years with a booster dose given at age 16 years.

- Administer one dose of MCV4 at ages 13 through 18 years if the child has not been vaccinated previously.

- Administer one dose to any college freshman living in a dormitory if he or she has never been vaccinated.

- Any child who has HIV should receive two doses of MCV4 at least eight weeks apart.

- Two doses of MCV4 should be administered at least eight weeks apart to children ages 2 through 10 years who have persistent complement component deficiency as well as asplenia (no spleen or a nonfunctioning spleen), followed by one dose every five years thereafter.

- Administer one dose of MCV4 to children ages 2 through 10 years who travel to countries with a high risk of meningococcal disease and during outbreaks caused by any of the serogroups. (Also see chapter 16, "Vaccines for Young Travelers.")

- Administer MCV4 to children who are at continued risk for meningococcal disease who had received a previous vaccination with MCV4 or MPSV4 after three years if the first dose they received was given at age 2 through 6 years.

## When to Delay or Avoid the Meningococcal Disease Vaccines

The CDC recommends that children who meet any of the following conditions should avoid getting the meningococcal vaccine: those who have had a life-threatening allergic reaction to a previous dose, those who have a life-threatening allergy to any of the ingredients in the vaccine, including latex that is present in the vial stopper, and those who have had Guillain-Barre syndrome. Vaccination should be delayed if your child has a moderate to severe illness at the time the immunization is scheduled.

## Side Effects of the Meningococcal Disease Vaccines

Side effects among the different meningococcal vaccines are somewhat similar but different enough to mention. The following figures about side effects are from studies reported in the individual vaccines' product information sheets.

For Menveo, the most common reactions among children ages 2 through 10 years include pain at the injection site (31 percent), redness of the skin (23 percent), irritability (18 percent), hardening of the skin (induration, 16 percent), sleepiness (14 percent), malaise (12 percent), and headache (11 percent). Adolescents and adults most often experience pain at the injection site (41 percent), headache (30 percent), muscle pain (18 percent), malaise (16 percent), and nausea (10 percent).

Among children at age 9 months given Menactra, reported side effects at the injection site include tenderness (37 percent), redness (30 percent), and swelling (17 percent). Other side effects include irritability (57 percent), abnormal crying (33 percent), loss of appetite (30 percent), drowsiness (30 percent), and vomiting (14 percent).

## CONCERNS AND CONTROVERSIES

If you are the parent of children age 11 to 16 years, have they received a meningococcal shot? If they got the first shot, did they get the booster? If you answered "no" to one or both of these questions, you could be in the majority, and that is a concern for public health officials. According to the results of a North Carolina survey published in May 2011, two-thirds of 1,281 parents of adolescents polled had knowledge of the meningococcal vaccine, but only 44 percent had had their children vaccinated. Another finding was that 39 percent of parents of unvaccinated adolescents said they probably or definitely would not have their children vaccinated in the next year. Note, however, that North Carolina is a state that does not require children to be immunized for meningococcal disease in order to enter school.

These statistics were presented at the 2011 annual meeting of the Society for Adolescent Health and Medicine by Dr. Tamera Coyne-Beasley, the lead investigator of the study and an associate professor of pediatrics and internal medicine at the University of North Carolina, Chapel Hill. She found that the main reason (25 percent) parents gave for not vaccinating their children was that their health-care provider had not recommended or mentioned the vaccine. Fourteen percent said their child did not need the vaccine, 9 percent were worried about vaccine safety, and 8 percent said they had not seen their doctor recently. However, most of the children (83 percent) had a regular health-care provider, 93 percent had health insurance, and 78 percent had had a preventive checkup in the past year.

This study is interesting for several reasons. First, as Dr. Coyne-Beasley concluded, "Awareness of a vaccine doesn't necessarily mean that one will get it." Second, one-quarter of health-care providers reportedly did not talk to parents about the vaccine. There could be a few reasons why doctors did not raise the topic with parents, including the fact that the vaccine is not mandated in North Carolina. Another interesting finding is that one-third of parents said they were not aware of the vaccine. That means a significant proportion of parents of adolescents eligible for the vaccine could not even make a decision about immunization because they were not aware the vaccine even existed.

The bottom line is that the vaccination process must

begin with awareness and education. Parents cannot help make decisions about their children's health if they don't have the information upon which to make a choice. Part of that information-sharing process should lie with health-care professionals and health-oriented organizations and institutions, and parents should be aware of the pros and cons, risks and benefits, of each vaccine before their child receives it.

# CHAPTER 14

Human Papillomavirus

In June 2011, the prestigious medical journal *The Lancet* published the results of a study showing the impact of administering the vaccine for human papillomavirus (HPV) to females aged 12 to 26 years. The study showed that the vaccine resulted in a nearly 50 percent reduction in precancerous abnormalities in the cervix in girls younger than 17 years old. However, the vaccine did not result in the same significant reduction in abnormalities in girls older than 17, an age when many females have already become sexually active and thus the vaccine is less likely to be protective.[1]

When the Centers for Disease Control and Prevention recommended immunizing girls as young as 11 years old for HPV, many eyebrows were raised, especially among parents, since HPV is a sexually transmitted disease. However, as the *Lancet* study indicates, there is more to the story: the HPV vaccine protects girls and young women against the types of HPV that can cause cancer, especially cervical cancer, and the vaccines are most effective if they are administered before individuals experience their first sexual contact. As for vaccinating young boys, this practice was recommended by the Advisory Committee on Immunization Practices of the CDC on October 24, 2011, and supported by the

American Academy of Pediatrics. HPV for males become part of the recommended immunization schedule in February 2012.

Immunization for HPV is the most recent addition to the recommended vaccination schedule, and so it is often the one parents know the least about and about which they have questions. This chapter will, I hope, clear up your questions about HPV and the vaccines developed to combat it.

## WHAT ARE HUMAN PAPILLOMAVIRUSES?

Human papillomaviruses (HPVs) are a group of 150 or more related viruses, of which about one-quarter can be transmitted via sexual activity. Many of the human papillomaviruses do not cause symptoms in people, but among those that do, some cause genital warts while others have the potential to cause cancer. Genital HPV is the most common sexually transmitted infection in the United States, affecting about 20 million Americans ages 15 to 49. More than half of sexually active people contract HPV at some point during their lifetime.

HPV can be low risk or high risk. The viruses that cause genital warts are considered low risk. Low-risk HPV infections often do not cause symptoms, and so most people never even know they are infected. When the infections cause symptoms, the infections often go away without any treatment over the course of a few years. The warts can take weeks, months, or even years to develop after sexual contact with an infected individual. In females the warts can grow in and around the outside of the vagina, on the vulva, cervix, or groin, and in or around the anus. In males, warts can develop on the penis, scrotum, thigh, or groin and in or around the anus. Rarely, genital warts grow in the mouth or throat if someone has had oral sex with an infected individual.

HPVs that can cause cancer are high risk. Having a high-risk HPV does not automatically lead to cancer. However, persistent infections with high-risk HPVs are the main cause of cervical cancer. Other cancers associated with HPVs include cervical, vulvar, vaginal, and anal cancer in women and anal and penile cancer in men.

## Symptoms of HPV

The only symptom of genital HPV is warts (bumps or clusters of bumps) in the genital area, but not everyone who has the disease develops the bumps. If they do appear, they usually develop within weeks or months after sexual contact with an infected person. If the warts are not treated, they may disappear, remain unchanged, or increase in size or number, but they will not turn into cancer.

Recurrent respiratory papillomatosis causes warts to grow in the throat. These growths may block the airway and cause hoarseness or difficulty breathing.

However, cervical cancer caused by high-risk HPV usually does not present any symptoms until it is advanced, which is why it is important for females to get screened for cervical cancer so it can be detected early. Other cancers related to HPV often do not have signs or symptoms until they are advanced as well.

## How HPV Is Transmitted

Genital HPV is transmitted by skin-to-skin and genital contact. In most cases it is passed during vaginal and anal sex. Much less frequently it is transmitted during oral sex or hand-to-genital contact. The viruses can be transmitted even when an infected person does not have any signs of symptoms of the disease. It is also possible to contract more than one type of HPV.

In rare cases, a pregnant woman who has genital HPV can pass the infection along to her infant during delivery. Children who contract HPV from their mother can develop juvenile-onset recurrent respiratory papillomatosis (JORRP), which, according to the RRP Foundation, develops in about twenty-three hundred children per year. JORRP is nearly always diagnosed by the time a child is 10 and usually before age 5 years. The disease is characterized by warty growths in the respiratory tract that can result in persistent hoarseness, difficulty speaking, loss of voice, and difficulty breathing.

## Risk Factors for HPV

Risk factors for genital HPV include:

- *Age.* Genital warts occur most often in adolescents and young adults.

- *Number of sexual partners.* The more sexual partners a person has, the more likely he or she is to contract a genital HPV infection.

- *Weak immune system.* Anyone who has a weakened immune system is at greater risk of acquiring HPV infections.

## Treatment of HPV

The good news about genital warts is that they usually disappear without treatment. However, even if the warts go away or have been removed, an individual can still harbor HPV and transmit the virus to other people.

Some of the medications used to eliminate warts are applied directly to the lesions and may require several applications before they disappear. Those medications include imiquimod (Aldara, Zyclara) and podofilox (Condylox), both of which are prescription drugs; and trichloroacetic acid, which is a chemical a doctor can use to burn off genital warts.

## ABOUT THE HPV VACCINES

The Food and Drug Administration has approved two vaccines, GARDASIL and CERVARIX, which are highly effective in preventing infection with the two HPV types (types 16 and 18) that are known to cause most cervical cancers, as well as vulvar, vaginal, and anal cancers. GARDASIL can also prevent infection with the two HPV types (types 6 and 11) that are responsible for most cases of genital warts. Therefore, GARDASIL is known as a quadivalent vaccine (HPV4), because it can help prevent cancers and genital warts caused by four different types of HPV. CERVARIX is a bivalent vaccine (HPV2), and it helps prevent cervical cancers in females.

Both vaccines are administered as shots and require three doses. Anyone who has already had sexual relations before receiving all three doses of an HPV vaccine may still benefit from getting the injections if he or she was not infected before vaccination with the HPV types in the vaccine. The most benefit from the HPV vaccine comes when individuals complete the three shot series before they begin sexual activity.

It's important to note that not all cervical, vulvar, vaginal, and anal cancers are caused by HPV and that neither vaccine protects against genital diseases not caused by HPV. Also, GARDASIL protects against only vulvar, vaginal, cervical, and anal cancers caused by HPV 16 and 18 and CERVARIX protects against only cervical cancers caused by HPV 16 and 18.

## GARDASIL

This HPV4 vaccine was licensed for use in June 2006 and is produced by Merck for intramuscular injection. The medium used during the fermentation process contains vitamins, amino acids, mineral salts, and carbohydrates. In addition to the four HPV-type proteins, each 0.5 mL dose of the vaccine contains approximately 225 mcg of aluminum hydroxyphosphate sulfate, 9.56 mg of sodium chloride, 0.78 mg of L-histidine (an amino acid), 50 mcg of polysorbate 80, 35 mcg of sodium borate, and less than 7 mcg of yeast protein. GARDASIL does not contain preservatives or antibiotics.

## CERVARIX

This HPV2 vaccine was licensed for use in 2009 and is produced by GlaxoSmithKline for intramuscular injection. Each 0.5 mL dose of the finished product contains the two HPV proteins plus 4.4 mg of sodium chloride, 0.624 mg of sodium dihydrogen phosphate dehydrate, and 0.5 mg of aluminum hydroxide, along with residual amounts of insect cell and viral protein (less than 40 ng) and bacterial cell protein (less than 150 ng) from the manufacturing process. CERVARIX does not contain any preservatives.

## Who Should Get the HPV Vaccine

HPV vaccines are recommended for 11- and 12-year-old males and females and for males and females ages 13 through 26 years old who did not receive any or all of the three recommended doses when they were younger. Two vaccines are available for this use—GARDASIL (HPV4) and CERVARIX (HPV2)—but only HPV4 is for use in males, while females can be given either HPV2 or HPV4.

Originally, the HPV vaccine was only recommended for females. However, after health authorities reviewed data showing the vaccine was effective in preventing genital warts in men and some cancers, including anal and oral cancers, the CDC recommended HPV vaccination for boys 11 to 12 years old and catch-up vaccination for those 13 to 18. Oral HPV is especially common among men.

## The HPV Schedule

The CDC recommends the following schedule for vaccination for HPV:

- First dose to females and males age 11 or 12 years

- Second dose one to two months after the first dose

- Third dose at least twenty-four weeks after the first dose

- Administer the series to females and males at ages 13 through 18 years if they have not been vaccinated previously.

## When to Delay or Avoid the HPV Vaccine

Sometimes the HPV vaccine should be delayed or avoided completely. Here are those times:

- If your child is pregnant, your health-care provider will likely advise against giving the vaccine unless it is clearly necessary.

- If your child is breast-feeding, your health-care provider may advise against giving the vaccine, because it is uncertain whether antibodies from the vaccine are excreted in breast milk.

## Side Effects of the HPV Vaccine

The most common side effects reported by females who receive the HPV vaccine are pain, swelling, and/or redness at the injection site, fever, nausea, dizziness, diarrhea, fatigue, headache, and muscle pain. Less common, but occurring in more than 1 percent of females, are joint pain, vomiting, cough, toothache, insomnia, stuffy nose, and generally not feeling well. Serious but rare side effects include a very high fever, an allergic reaction, Guillain-Barre syndrome (characterized by weakness, tingling, or paralysis), gastroenteritis (inflammation of the stomach and intestines, usually involving diarrhea or vomiting), pelvic inflammatory disease, asthma or bronchospasms, blood clots in the lungs or legs, seizures, and appendicitis.

There has been some controversy surrounding side

effects associated with GARDASIL, including deaths among females. See "Concerns and Controversies" for more details.

## CONCERNS AND CONTROVERSIES

The HPV vaccine is the subject of several controversies, and not only because it is a vaccine administered to young people for a disease that is transmitted through sexual contact; cost and safety also are part of the debate. Here are some of the issues that have been raised.

### Cost Concerns

In October 2010, the CDC began to reconsider the question of whether it should recommend young males be vaccinated with the HPV vaccine, to protect against not only human wart virus but also a number of cancers.

Dr. Lauri Markowitz, who heads the ACIP's HPV working group, noted that the number of cases of cancer is rising in the United States, especially among women and men who have sex with men. She also stated that many feel administering the vaccine to adolescent males before they become sexually active—and without requiring them to reveal their sexual orientation—is the best way to protect them against cancers associated with HPV.

In addition, CDC researchers and vaccine experts told a meeting of the ACIP that the vaccine is safe and cost-effective, but some advisors are worried that the $360 cost is too high.[2]

### Safety Concerns

All vaccines are associated with side effects, but some raise more concern than others. Such may be the case with GARDASIL. Between the time the vaccine was licensed in June

2006 and February 14, 2011, approximately 33 million doses of GARDASIL had been distributed in the United States. During that time, the Vaccine Adverse Event Reporting System (VAERS) received 18,354 reports of adverse events that followed vaccination.

Overall, 92 percent of the reported events were classified as nonserious, which the VAERS defines as events other than hospitalization, death, permanent disability, or life-threatening illness. Thus nonserious events included symptoms such as fainting, headache, nausea, fever, pain, and swelling at the injection site.

As with all VAERS reports, the serious events reported may or may not have been caused by the vaccine. In the case of GARDASIL, there were 51 VAERS reports of death among females as of February 14, 2011. Among males who received GARDASIL there were 205 VAERS reports, of which 15 were serious and 2 of the 15 were deaths.

Back in 2009, the *Journal of the American Medical Association* published a study in which it noted the number of adverse events following immunization with HPV from June 1, 2006, through December 31, 2008. At that time there were 12,424 reports of adverse events, with 772 (6.2 percent) being categorized as serious, including 32 reports of death. The study's authors also pointed out a "disproportional reporting of syncope [fainting] and venous thromboembolic events [blood clots]" associated with the vaccine compared with other vaccines.

This article appeared with an editorial by Charlotte Haug, MD, PhD, MSc, titled "The Risks and Benefits of HPV Vaccination," in which the author presents some important food for thought for parents. Briefly, Haug notes that while the theory behind the HPV vaccine is "sound," "in practice the issue is more complex." One issue is that the vaccine targets only two cancer-causing strains while "at least 15 of them are oncogenic." Another point is that "the relationship between infection at a young age and development of cancer 20 to 40 years later is not known" and that "it is impossible to predict exactly what effect vaccination of young girls and women will have on the incidence of cervical cancer 20 to 40 years from now."

# CHAPTER 15

Action Plan: How to Individualize Your Child's
Vaccination Schedule

Now that you have had a chance to review all the vaccines
and the controversies, as well as the safety issues, you may
be thinking, *Now that I have this information, what steps do
I need to take to ensure my child is protected from these?*

This chapter introduces you to some options parents have
to individualize their child's vaccination schedule, as well as
the steps to take should you need help implementing your
plan and/or your child experiences any adverse reactions to
vaccines.

This chapter is complete with contact information, Web
sites, and other relevant tidbits parents and caregivers can use
to help ensure they have what they need to make informed
decisions about vaccinating their children. When Web site
URLs are provided, I recommend you visit the sites and re-
check any contact and other relevant information: contact information, like the world of vaccines, is ever changing.

## ALTERNATIVE VACCINATION SCHEDULES

Many parents, as well as a number of physicians, question
the safety of exposing infants and young children to multiple

vaccines because of concerns about increasing their risk of developing side effects or adverse reactions. One way to address these concerns is to turn to an alternative vaccination schedule.

An alternative vaccination schedule is not the same as the CDC's approved catch-up schedule (see appendices), which is designed to show physicians and parents how they can "catch up" when a child falls behind in receiving his or her recommended vaccines. Alternative or selective vaccination schedules are not approved or reviewed by the CDC or any other public health organization. Instead, they are schedules developed by physicians who believe that the CDC model may not always serve the best needs of children and that alternatives should be available and offered to parents so they can make an informed decision about immunization.

Parents who seek out alternative vaccination schedules are typically those who are concerned about giving their children one or more specific vaccines or giving their child more than one vaccine at a time (even though the CDC says administering multiple vaccines is safe) or who want to otherwise customize their child's vaccination schedule for his or her needs. Several physicians have shared their alternative vaccination schedules. Here are several for you to consider. Also discuss an alternative vaccination schedule with a knowledgeable physician.

I want to point out, however, that although here I discuss only a few doctors who have alternative vaccination schedules, there are a growing number of doctors who are very willing to work with parents and children to develop alternative plans. In fact, a recent study illustrates this very idea. Is your doctor one of them?

In a study appearing in the May 2011 issue of the *American Journal of Preventive Medicine,* researchers from the University of Colorado School of Medicine surveyed nearly seven hundred pediatricians and family medicine physicians and found that a growing number of parents are asking doctors to spread out vaccines. The researchers noted that 20 percent of the doctors said at least 10 percent of parents make the request and 64 percent of all physicians said they agreed to spread out vaccines in the primary series at least sometimes. In the same survey, 8 percent of the doctors said that at least 10 percent of parents refused a vaccine at some point.

## Dr. Robert Sears

The most well-known example of an alternative vaccination schedule is the one developed by Dr. Robert Sears, author of *The Vaccine Book: Making the Right Decision for Your Child*. The Sears schedule spreads out the vaccinations over a longer time span (up to age 5 to 6 years) and arranges the vaccines in a different order based on how common and severe the diseases are, and he recommends not giving children more than two vaccines at the same time. To address the fears of parents who are most reluctant to vaccinate their children, his schedule includes what he calls the "bare minimum" vaccinations, and it also omits polio.

According to Sears' book, his alternative vaccination schedule "does eventually provide complete protection from diseases, and it does so at an age-appropriate pace. It gives kids protection from diseases at the ages when those diseases are the most troublesome, and it doesn't necessarily overload young kids with vaccines that they don't really need until they're older."

For example, Sears suggests that parents who are not comfortable having their children get the MMR shot at age 12 months "could safely delay the vaccine until your child enters school, since he is unlikely to come into contact with anyone who has one of these three illnesses." Dr. Sears acknowledges that not vaccinating your children does increase their risk of developing disease. He emphasizes, however, that he is willing to work with worried parents who would rather risk the disease than any risk associated with the vaccine.

The argument defending the CDC's recommended schedule is that although infants are born with protection from their mothers from diseases, the protection begins to fade

after birth and immunizing infants in the first six months of
life stimulates the immune system so babies can begin making their own antibodies while they are losing the benefits
from their mothers' antibodies.

## Kenneth Bock, MD

Another advocate of an alternative vaccination schedule is
Kenneth Bock, MD, author of *Healing the New Childhood
Epidemics: Autism, ADHD, Asthma, and Allergies.* The
most striking difference in Dr. Bock's schedule is for hepatitis B: he recommends the first dose shortly before starting
day care. (Babies born to hepatitis B positive mothers, however, should get the vaccine at birth.) For children who do
not attend day care, he recommends postponing the vaccination until the year before kindergarten. The second dose
should come one to two months after the first, and the third
should be given four to six months after the second.

Generally, Dr. Bock's alternative schedule involves delaying immunization: for example, he suggests administering the first doses of Hib and of polio at age 4 months
instead of age 2 months. He also suggests the first dose of
DTaP be given at age 5 months instead of age 2 months and
the pneumococcal vaccine be delayed until age 2 years instead of 2 months of age, by which time your child will need
only one dose instead of four.

- Hib: first dose at 4 months, second at 6 months,
  third at 8 months, and fourth at 17 months of age.

- Polio: First dose at 4 months, second dose at
  6 months, third at 17 months, and booster at ages 4
  to 6 years.

- DTaP: first dose at 5 months, second dose at 7
  months, third dose at 9 months, fourth dose at 18
  months, and booster at ages 4 to 5 years.

- Pneumococcal: one dose only, at age 2 years.

- Varicella: one dose at age 4 to 5 years, if mandated by law and if your child does not have evidence of immunity.

- MMR: measles at 15 months old, rubella at 6 to 12 months after measles, mumps at 6 to 12 months after rubella. Boosters should be given separately at age 4 to 5 years. Check your child's titers before making the appointment for the boosters, and if your child shows immunity no booster will be necessary.

To accompany your child's vaccination program, Dr. Bock recommends supplements for children who are old enough to take them and who have no history of reactions to them. Vitamins A (preferably as cod-liver oil) and C, along with zinc and transfer factor, are recommended to be given one to two weeks before the vaccination, on the day of vaccination, and for two weeks after. Dosages should be appropriate for your child's age, size, and health status. Other physicians offer alternative vaccination schedules, including Stephanie Cave, MD, and Donald W. Miller, Jr., MD. But given that 64 percent of physicians in the recent survey said they agreed to spread out vaccines at least sometimes means your chances are pretty good there is a pediatrician in your area—perhaps even your pediatrician—who will work with you on establishing an alternative vaccination schedule that is best for your son or daughter.

## FINDING THE RIGHT PEDIATRICIAN

Do you and your pediatrician see eye-to-eye on the issue of vaccinations? If the answer is "no," now is the time to make a choice: is your physician willing to work with you to establish a vaccination program for your child that is agreeable to you,

### DOCTORS REFUSING TO TREAT UNVACCINATED CHILDREN

In March 2011, several news agencies reported about a practice among a growing number of physicians: those who refuse to care for children whose parents elect not to vaccinate their youngsters. The reports were based on interviews with physicians across the United States. The reports reflected that (1) while more parents are making efforts to find doctors who have a philosophy about vaccinations that matches theirs, (2) there are also physicians who are turning away children when their parents will not have them vaccinated.

The most recent study (2005) to examine this issue was published in the *Archives of Pediatric and Adolescent Medicine*. A total of 1,004 randomly selected members of the American Academy of Pediatrics were surveyed, of whom 39 percent said they would stop treating a family that refused all vaccinations, while 28 percent said they would dismiss a family if it refused select vaccines. An earlier survey done by the American Academy of Pediatrics in 2001, found that 23 percent of doctors "always" or "sometimes" told parents they would no longer be their child's physician if the parents refused to give their children the proper vaccinations.

or is it time for you to move on and find a physician whose philosophy is similar to yours?

Parents who challenge the conventional childhood vaccination schedules run the risk of alienating their pediatrician. If your philosophy about vaccinations does not match your doctor's and the issue cannot be resolved, it is best to know this as soon as possible so you can shop around for another physician for your child. If your current doctor cannot provide you with a referral, you can contact a children's hospital in your area, the American Academy of Pediatrics, the Holistic Pediatric Association, the American College for Advancement in Medicine, or the American Holistic Medical Association for assistance in locating a like-minded physician in your area. (See the appendices.)

## VACCINE EXEMPTIONS AND HOW TO GET THEM

Although there is no federal law mandating vaccinations, all fifty states have their own laws that require children to be vaccinated against some or all of the following diseases before attending public school or state-licensed day-care facilities: diphtheria, measles, mumps, pertussis, polio, rubella, and tetanus. In addition, all fifty states also provide at least one type of exemption to this rule. As of 2011, all the states offered medical exemptions, forty-eight offered an exemption for religious reasons, and twenty allowed an exemption for philosophical beliefs. When you factor in all three exemptions, only two states—Mississippi and West Virginia—offer only a medical exemption.

Because each state has its own statutes on regulations and exemptions, you need to contact the state board of health, the department of public health, or whatever other entity in your state is responsible for regulating vaccinations to learn more about exemptions for your child. Some states specifically include private schools in their requirements, although most private schools have similar or identical requirements for their students. If you homeschool your child, he or she is generally not subject to the state's vaccination requirements. As of 2010, the only state that required vaccination of homeschooled children was North Carolina.

## ACCESS TO INDIVIDUAL STATE VACCINATION EXEMPTION INFORMATION

Institute for Vaccine Safety: http://www.vaccinesafety
.edu/cc-exem.htm

National Vaccine Information Center: http://www.nvic
.org/Vaccine-Laws/state-vaccine-requirements
.aspx

ProCon: http://vaccines.procon.org/view.resource.php
?resourceID=003597

If you move to another state after your child enters school and you have an exemption, you will need to inquire about the validity of your exemption in your new state and you may need to reapply. Children who have not received all their required vaccinations or a valid exemption are not allowed to attend school, although each state enforces any breach of the law in different ways. If there is an outbreak of disease covered by vaccinations, children who have an exemption will be barred from attending school.

Here is some basic information about the three types of vaccination exemptions.

## Medical Exemption

All fifty states provide for a medical exemption, but the process differs from state to state. If you seek a medical exemption for your child because he or she cannot receive a vaccine out of safety concerns, the first thing you should do is apply well in advance of the school year, as states receive many applications for exemptions each year. If the school year arrives and you have a pending application, most schools will not allow your child to enroll until he or she has either the vaccinations or an exemption letter.

Proof of a medical exemption must be a signed statement by an MD or OD (doctor of osteopathy) stating that administration of one or more vaccines to a child would be detrimental to his or her health. While some states will accept a private physician's written exemption statement, others require a review by the state's health department, which can refuse the request if officials do not think the exemption is justified.

## Religious Exemption

All states except Mississippi and West Virginia offer a religious exemption. If you are wondering what the difference is between a philosophical or personal belief exemption and a religious exemption, the answer is, it is often ambiguous. Some states are specific, using language that says an objection to a vaccine must be based on the tenets of a specific, organized religion and the parent must be a member of a bona fide religion that has written tenets that prohibit invasive medical procedures such as vaccination. Some states require parents to get a signed affidavit from their pastor or spiritual advisor that affirms their sincere religious belief concerning vaccinations.

Other states use more general terms regarding a religious exemption, such as "a sincere and meaningful belief . . . held with the strength of traditional religious convictions." This could be interpreted as a personal philosophical belief.

If you seek a religious exemption, carefully review the requirements for your state and be prepared to be challenged. If your request is challenged, you could be required to prove your religious beliefs in court. The religious exemption is based on the First Amendment; therefore, a state must have a "compelling State interest" to refuse a citizen's right to freely exercise his or her religion. However, a state can say that the possibility of spreading a communicable disease is a "compelling State interest" and deny the exemption. Therefore, if you belong to a church it is advisable to get a letter from your spiritual leader that affirms your religious beliefs.

## Philosophical Belief Exemption

A philosophical belief exemption, also known as a personal belief exemption, is available in twenty states. As of April 16, 2009, the states that offered this exemption were Arizona, Arkansas, California, Colorado, Idaho, Louisiana, Maine, Michigan, Minnesota, New Mexico, North Dakota, Ohio, Oklahoma, Oregon, Pennsylvania, Texas, Utah, Vermont, Washington, and Wisconsin.

Parents who seek an exemption on philosophical grounds frequently say it is their right to decide which medical care their children will receive without the government getting involved. However, the U.S. Supreme Court has ruled in some cases that state vaccination requirements are permissible, explaining that "the very concept of ordered liberty precludes allowing every person to make his own standards on matters of conduct in which the society as a whole has important interests."

In many of the twenty states, in order to use the philosophical belief exemption you must object to all vaccines, not just a specific one. The future of this exemption is questionable, as federal health officials and medical organizations are asking state legislators to eliminate it. Be sure to check the status of the philosophical belief exemption in your state if you wish to use it.

## Proof of Existing Immunity

Another exemption option open to parents is proof of existing immunity. Some states will allow exemptions to certain vaccines if you show proof your child already has immunity to the disease(s), which typically occurs because a child has already had the disease and thus developed antibodies against it. Check with your state laws to see which vaccines in your state can be exempted if you can provide proof of immunity.

To get proof of immunity, you can go to a private medical laboratory and have your child undergo a blood test to see if there are enough antibodies to provide immunity to a disease such as measles or whooping cough. If the antibody levels are within accepted standards, you may be able to use this proof of immunity to get an exemption to vaccination. Insurance may or may not cover such tests, and the cost for the necessary blood tests varies, depending on the disease.

## HOW TO REPORT ADVERSE REACTIONS

What should you do if your child experiences an adverse reaction to a vaccine? Naturally, the first thing you will do is attend to the symptoms by providing relief and/or contacting your pediatrician. But the next thing you should do is report the event to the Vaccine Adverse Event Reporting System, with the help of your physician. (Physicians are strongly encouraged, although not required, to report adverse reactions to vaccines.) VAERS is a passive safety surveillance program, which means it collects information—but does not act on it—about possible side effects that occur after someone has received a vaccine licensed for use in the United States. The program is cosponsored by the Centers for Disease Control and Prevention and the Food and Drug Administration.

VAERS receives about thirty thousand reports each year, of which 13 percent (thirty-nine hundred) are classified as serious; that is, the adverse reaction involves disability, hospitalization, life-threatening illness, or death. The remainder of the reports include mild to moderate events, including fever, crying, irritability, poor feeding, and diarrhea.

If you are not sure if you should report a specific side effect or even if it is related to the vaccine, remember that VAERS encourages the reporting of any clinically significant adverse event that happens after a vaccine is administered. You do not need to make the report all alone: in fact, you are encouraged to seek help from your health-care professional in filling out the VAERS form. Only about 7 percent of vaccine recipients, including their parents or guardians, send in reports. By submitting a report you can help VAERS monitor and identify any important new safety issues, which in turn allows them to assist in the pursuit of additional research that may result in changes in vaccine recommendations.

Most VAERS reports are submitted by vaccine manufacturers (37 percent) and health-care providers (36%). The National Childhood Vaccine Injury Act (NCVIA) requires health-care providers to report any adverse event that is listed by a vaccine manufacturer as a contraindication to further doses of the vaccine, and any adverse event listed in the VAERS Table of Reportable Events Following Vaccination that occurs within the amount of time specified after vaccination. The list and relevant events by vaccine can be accessed at the following address: http://vaers.hhs.gov/re sources/VAERS_Table_of_Reportable_Events_Following _Vaccination.pdf.


## THE VACCINE INJURY COMPENSATION PROGRAM

I hope you never need to seek compensation for injuries related to a vaccine, but if you do, there is a program you can use. In 1986, the National Childhood Vaccine Injury Act of 1986 (the Act) was created by Congress. This act acknowledged that

- vaccines can cause injuries,

- people injured by vaccines and their families should be compensated financially, and

- vaccine safety protections are needed to be part of the mass vaccination system.

This law established the National Vaccine Injury Compensation Program (NVICP), a program available to help you and your child should he or she ever be injured by a vac-

## COMPENSATION DENIED: THE BRUESEWITZ CASE

In February 2011, the U.S. Supreme Court ruled in favor of vaccine manufacturers in a case brought by Russell and Robalee Bruesewitz, who challenged the National Childhood Vaccine Injury Act. The Bruesewitzes' child, Hannah, experienced seizures and subsequently suffered developmental problems after receiving the third of five scheduled doses of Wyeth's Tri-Immunol diphtheria-pertussis-tetanus vaccine in 1992. The vaccine is no longer sold. (Wyeth is now part of Pfizer.)

Hannah requires specialized care for the rest of her life. When her parents originally filed a claim to the vaccine court, the severe injuries Hannah reportedly suffered were eliminated from the qualifying list for compensation one month before her case was heard. When their claim was rejected in vaccine court, the Bruesewitz family pursued their claim at the federal level.

In the 6-2 decision, the Supreme Court justices said that the National Childhood Vaccine Injury Act of 1986 preempted claims by the Bruesewitz family that the vaccine manufacturer knew at the time there was a safer vaccine for diphtheria-tetanus-pertussis but did not produce it. That federal law was designed to encourage vaccine production by limiting lawsuits by patients. Instead, it channels most complaints into a no-fault system funded by vaccine manufacturers that offers limited but guaranteed compensation for injuries that are shown to be caused by a vaccine.

If the ruling had gone in favor of the Bruesewitz family, it would have opened the door for other parents who said vaccines had caused autism to sue vaccine makers.

Two justices dissented—Sonia Sotomayor and Ruth Bader Ginsburg—and the former stated that the ruling "leaves a regulatory vacuum in which no one ensures that vaccine manufacturers adequately take account of scientific and technological advancements when designing or distributing their products." The American Academy of Pediatrics, however, agreed with the ruling. President O. Marion Burton stated that the court's decision "protects children by strengthening our national immunization system and ensuring that vaccines will continue to prevent the spread of infectious diseases in this country."

cine. The NVICP is administered by the Health Resources and Services Administration, and according to the NVICP Web site, it was established "to ensure an adequate supply of vaccines, stabilize vaccine costs, and establish and maintain an accessible and efficient forum for individuals found to be injured by certain vaccines," and those vaccines are those recommended by the CDC for routine use.

The U.S. Court of Federal Claims makes the decisions about who will be paid regarding vaccine injury claims, and three federal government offices work together to administer the NVICP: the U.S. Department of Health and Human Services, the U.S. Department of Justice, and the U.S. Court of Federal Claims.

The Act preserves the right for anyone injured by a vaccine to bring a lawsuit in the court system if they are denied federal compensation or if it is not sufficient. By 2010, the U.S. Court of Claims had awarded more than $2 billion to victims of vaccines. This amount represents only one-third of people who applied for such compensation; two-thirds of applicants have been denied. (For an example of a case that was denied compensation, see "Compensation Denied: The Bruesewitz Case.")

## TO CONTACT THE NVICP

1-800-338-2382

Web site: http://www.hrsa.gov/vaccinecompensation
/default.htm

How to file a claim: http://www.hrsa.gov/vaccinecom
pensation/fileclaim.html

Parents should also be aware of the legal requirements set forth by the Act for vaccine providers. Your vaccine provider should:

- Provide you with risk and benefit information for each vaccine before your child is vaccinated

- Keep written records of the manufacturers' names and the lot numbers of each vaccination given

- Note any serious health problems that follow vaccination on your child's permanent medical record

- Report serious health problems that follow vaccination to VAERS

The NVICP and VAERS are not connected; submitting a report to VAERS in no way notifies or intersects with the NVICP. Therefore, you must file a separate form with each program.

# CHAPTER 16

Vaccines for Young Travelers

If you are planning to take your children on a trip outside the United States, one item you may need to put on your "To Do" list is to check on vaccination requirements. While you can take a vacation in Canada or Bermuda without getting any vaccinations, a jaunt to Mexico, Egypt, the Philippines, or Turkey is a different story. When you and your family go away on holiday, the last thing you want to bring home with you along with souvenirs is a chronic or life-threatening disease. You can avoid such unwelcome surprises if you are prepared.

This chapter discusses the various vaccines your children may need when traveling out of the United States, as well as some tips for preventing disease when going abroad.

## PLANNING FOR TRAVEL VACCINATIONS

Long before you pack your suitcases, check to see if there are any vaccinations your children (and you) will need. To help you with this process, here are some steps you should take:

- Make sure your children (and you) are up to date with vaccinations recommended by the CDC. Even though the diseases associated with these vaccines do not occur often in the United States, they are still common in many parts of the world. If your child will be out of the country when he or she is due for one or more recommended vaccines, you and your doctor may need to discuss adjusting your child's immunization schedule.

- Check with the CDC or a knowledgeable physician (e.g., your pediatrician or a travel doctor) to determine which vaccinations may be needed for the locations you and your children will visit. (The CDC site is: http://wwwnc.cdc.gov/travel/destinations/list.htm.) The only vaccinations that are *required* by the International Health Regulations is for yellow fever if you are traveling to certain countries in sub-Saharan Africa and tropical South America. The meningococcal vaccination is required by the Saudi Arabian government for annual travel during the hajj. Otherwise, all other vaccinations are either routine (i.e., the routine childhood vaccinations) or recommended. The CDC notes which vaccines are recommended in specific countries to protect travelers from illnesses that occur in other areas of the world and to prevent people from transporting infectious diseases across international borders.

- Make an appointment with your physician to get the necessary vaccines. Ideally, make the appointment for up to four to six weeks before you leave on your trip, as most vaccines take time to become effective and some vaccines must be given in a series over days or weeks.

- If you and your child are traveling to a country or region that requires yellow fever vaccination, you will need to locate a clinic in your area that can administer the vaccination and issue a yellow fever certificate. To find which countries require a yellow fever vaccination and certification, you can access the CDC site at: http://wwwnc.cdc.gov/travel /yellowbook/2010/chapter-2/yellow-fever-vaccine -requirements-and-recommendations.htm. A resource to find a clinic is offered by the CDC at: http://wwwnc.cdc.gov/travel/yellow-fever-vaccina tion-clinics/search.htm. For information on Saudi Arabia's requirements, see: http://wwwnc.cdc.gov /travel/destinations/saudi-arabia.htm.

## VACCINES FIRST, THEN BON VOYAGE!

The following vaccines are required or recommended when traveling internationally: vaccines for yellow fever, Japanese encephalitis, and typhoid fever. However, because there are additional precautions you should know concerning some of the routine childhood vaccinations when traveling, that information is provided here as well.

## YELLOW FEVER

Yellow fever is a viral disease that is transmitted to people when they are bitten by infected mosquitoes. Areas of the world most inhabited by infected mosquitoes include tropical regions of Africa and parts of South America. Although yellow fever is very rare among U.S. travelers and the last epidemic in North America was more than a century ago in 1905 in New Orleans, vaccination against the disease is required in some countries.

### Symptoms

Symptoms of yellow fever can range from mild to severe and include high fever, chills, headache, muscle aches, vomiting, and backache. Complications can include bleeding, shock, and kidney and liver failure. Severe cases can be fatal.

There is no specific treatment for yellow fever. Symptoms can be relieved using rest, fluids, and medications such as ibuprofen, acetaminophen, or naproxen.

## How to Safeguard Against Yellow Fever

You and your children should take precautions against mosquito bites when traveling in areas where yellow fever is a problem. In addition to vaccination, here are some tips:

- Use an insect repellent that does not contain DEET (N,N-diethyl-m-toulamide). Instead, look for items that contain oil of lemon eucalyptus or one that contains two or more of the following oils: citronella, cinnamon, castor, rosemary, lemongrass, cedar, peppermint, clove, geranium.

- Wear protective clothing (long sleeves, long pants, socks, shoes). You can also treat clothing with the insecticide permethrin.

- Avoid being outside when mosquitoes are most active, especially at dusk and dawn.

- Use mosquito netting when sleeping, especially for infants and young children.

- Avoid using items that have a fragrance, such as shampoos, body lotions, and soaps.

## Vaccine

The yellow fever vaccine is called YF-VAX, and it is made by Sanofi Pasteur. The live, attenuated vaccine is prepared using chicken embryos, and each 0.5 mL subcutaneous dose contains sorbitol, gelatin, and sodium chloride. No preservatives are used, but the stopper of the vial contains latex.

Side effects associated with yellow fever vaccine include mild headache, muscle aches, low-grade fever, or other minor symptoms for five to ten days. Pain, swelling, and hypersensitivity at the injection site are also common. The manufacturer warns that no infant younger than 9 months should receive the vaccine because of an increased risk of encephalitis. If it is necessary for your infant to travel in an area where yellow fever is endemic, consult your physician.

## JAPANESE ENCEPHALITIS

Japanese encephalitis is a virus that is transmitted by mosquitoes. Travelers to Asia are at risk for this disease, which can be seasonal in temperate parts of Asia but year-round in more tropical climates. The risk of contracting Japanese encephalitis is low if you and your children stay a short time in Asia, but long-term travelers should be vaccinated.

Japanese encephalitis is very rare in the United States, with fewer than one case per year reported in U.S. civilians and military personnel who travel to and who are living in Asia. In Asia, however, thirty to fifty thousand cases are reported each year.

### Symptoms

Mild infections of Japanese encephalitis typically have no symptoms other than fever with headache. People who develop more severe infection can experience a headache that comes on quickly, high fever, neck stiffness, disorientation, tremors, convulsions (especially infants), stupor, and coma. The mortality rate ranges from 0.3 to 60 percent.

## Vaccines

Two vaccines have been developed for Japanese encephalitis for use in the United States:

- *JE-VAX* has been licensed in the United States since 1992 for travelers age 1 year and older. Production of JE-VAX was discontinued in 2006, and Sanofi Pasteur has reserved all remaining supplies for children ages 1 to 16 years old, because the newer vaccine, IXIARO, is not licensed for younger people. JE-VAX is an inactivated vaccine prepared using infected mouse brain. In addition to the viral strain, each 1.0 mL dose (which is for persons 3 years of age and older) contains about 500 mcg of gelatin, less than 100 mcg of formaldehyde, less than 0.0007 percent polysorbate 80, less than 50 ng of mouse serum protein, and 0.007 percent thimerosal. The 0.5 mL single dose is for children ages 1 to 3 years. The recommended primary immunization series is three doses: the second dose should be given seven days after the first, and the third should be administered thirty days after the first. The last dose should be given at least ten days before beginning international travel to make sure the body can build an adequate immune response.

- *IXIARO* (Intercell Biomedical) was approved by the FDA in March 2009 for people age 17 years and older. IXIARO is administered via intramuscular injection and requires two doses, twenty-eight days apart. Both doses should be completed at least one week before potential exposure. Each 0.5 mL dose of the inactivated vaccine contains 250 mcg of aluminum hydroxide, formaldehyde (not more than 200 pg/mL), sodium metabisulphite (not more than 200 ppm), and protamine sulfate (not more than 1 ug/mL). No antibiotics, preservatives, or stabilizers are present in the vaccine.

The most common side effects are swelling, pain, and/or tenderness at the injection site, affecting up to 30 percent of vaccines. About 10 percent of people experience fever, headache, malaise, rash, chills, dizziness, nausea, vomiting, and abdominal pain.

## TYPHOID FEVER

Typhoid fever is a life-threatening illness caused by the bacterium *Salmonella enterica* serotype Typhi. About 22 million cases of typhoid fever occur each year around the world, and two hundred thousand people die of the disease. The area of the world where travelers are at greatest risk is Southeast Asia, which also has a high risk of infections that are resistant to antibiotic treatment. Other areas of the world at high risk for infections are East Asia, Africa, the Caribbean, and Central and South America.

In the United States, about four hundred cases are reported each year, and 75 percent of them are acquired while traveling internationally. Therefore, protecting your children and yourself against typhoid fever is important if you are traveling in certain areas of the world.

### Symptoms

Symptoms of typhoid fever include a persistent fever as high as 103 to 104°F, along with weakness, stomach pains, headache, and loss of appetite. A rose-colored rash occurs in some patients. Constipation is common in older children and adults, while diarrhea may affect younger children. Less common complications include intestinal perforation, hemorrhage, and death. A diagnosis is confirmed using a stool or blood test.

## How to Safeguard Against Typhoid

Typhoid fever is spread mainly by consuming water or food that has been contaminated by feces from an infected individual or a carrier who has no symptoms. The main ways to protect your children and yourself against typhoid fever when going to regions of intermediate or high risk are the following:

- Drink bottled water or water that has been boiled for at least one minute before you drink it. Carbonated water is safer than uncarbonated water.

- Avoid drinks that contain ice or flavored ices that may have been made with contaminated water.

- If you eat raw fruits and vegetables, peel them yourself and wash them with uncontaminated water.

- Do not eat food or drink beverages from street vendors.

- Eat foods that have been cooked thoroughly and while they are still hot.

- Avoid fruits and vegetables that cannot be peeled. Greens are especially susceptible to contamination because they are difficult to clean.

## Vaccines

Currently there are two vaccines available in the United States for typhoid fever. Both protect 50 to 80 percent of people who receive them.

- *Vivotif,* an oral live, attenuated vaccine (made by Crucell/Berna). This vaccine is not recommended for children younger than 6 years of age. Primary vaccination with Vivotif consists of four capsules, and you must take one every other day about one hour before a meal. The entire series should be completed one week before potential exposure. A booster dose is necessary after five years if continued protection is needed.

- *Typhim Vi,* a polysaccharide vaccine (made by Sanofi Pasteur) given by injection. The main vaccination with Typhim Vi consists of a single injection given at least two weeks before expected exposure. Sanofi Pasteur does not recommend this vaccine for infants and children younger than 2 years of age. A booster dose is necessary after two years if continued protection is needed. Each 0.5 mL dose is formulated to contain 4.15 mg of sodium chloride, 0.065 mg of disodium phosphate, and 0.023 mg of monosodium phosphate.

As a parent, you should know the following about the typhoid vaccines:

- The live, attenuated vaccine should not be given to a child who is immunocompromised, including those who are infected with HIV. The injected vaccine theoretically is a safer alternative.

- Children who are experiencing a fever should not receive either vaccine until they have recovered. Neither vaccine should be given to any child who has a history of severe local or systemic reactions to a previous dose.

- Do not assume just because your child has been vaccinated against typhoid fever that he or she will be protected from the disease. The vaccines are not completely effective, so it is critical to be careful about which foods and beverages your child consumes when traveling in risky areas.

## TRAVEL-RELATED TIPS FOR ROUTINE VACCINATIONS

Some routine childhood vaccinations have some special travel-related information you should know about before traveling with your children. Here are some tips to consider.

### Hib

- If your child is younger than 15 months and has not been vaccinated for Hib, he or she should receive at least two doses before travel. The interval between doses can be as short as four weeks.

- Unvaccinated infants and children ages 15 to 59 months should receive a single dose of Hib before travel.

- Children older than 59 months do not need to be vaccinated unless they have a specific medical condition (e.g., immunodeficiency, immunosuppression, no spleen).

### MMR

- If your child is age 6 to 11 months and must travel outside the United States, he or she should receive the MMR vaccine before departure. Unfortunately, no single vaccines (monovalent) for measles, mumps, or rubella are available in the United States.

## Meningococcal

- The Saudi Arabian government requires meningo-coccal vaccination when traveling to Mecca during the annual hajj.

- The CDC recommends travelers be vaccinated before traveling to sub-Saharan Africa during the dry season (December through June) because epidemics are known to occur during this time.

## Hepatitis A

Hepatitis A is one of the diseases in the CDC's list of recommended vaccinations for children. It is also a disease that can be contracted in many foreign countries. Health-care providers should administer an injection for hepatitis A for anyone who travels for any reason, frequency, or duration to countries that have a high or intermediate risk of HAV infection. Generally, there is a high prevalence of antibody to hepatitis A virus in Mexico, Central and South America, Africa, Asia, the Middle East, India, and Greenland. The CDC has noted that most travel-related cases (72 percent) of hepatitis A have been associated with travel to Mexico or Central/South America.

Always check with the CDC's Travelers' Health information (Web site: http://wwwnc.cdc.gov/travel/) and with a knowledgeable physician for hepatitis A vaccine requirements as you plan your trip, as the prevalence status can change at any time anywhere in the world. According to the CDC:

- All susceptible persons who plan to travel to countries that have high or intermediate hepatitis A endemicity should receive the hepatitis A vaccination or immunoglobulin before leaving the United States. The first dose of hepatitis A vaccine should be administered as soon as you know your child will be traveling.

- One dose of monovalent hepatitis A vaccine given any time before leaving the United States can provide adequate protection for most healthy individuals younger than 40 years old.

- For long-term protection, it is necessary to complete the vaccine series.

- For children younger than 12 months of age or for children who cannot or have not received the vaccine, a single dose of immunoglobulin should be given. This dose will provide protection for up to three months, after which the child will need another dose.

- If administered within two weeks of exposure to hepatitis A virus, immunoglobulin is more than 85 percent effective in preventing HAV infection.

To help prevent infection with hepatitis A while traveling, you and your child should take the following precautions:

- Avoid dairy products.

- Do not eat any raw or undercooked fish or meat.

- Handle fresh fruits and vegetables yourself to make sure they are not washed in contaminated water.

- Do not consume food from street vendors.

- Use only bottled water for drinking and brushing your teeth.

- If you do not have access to bottled water, boil other water for at least one minute to make it safe to drink.

## Hepatitis B

Hepatitis B, which is covered in chapter 3, has an intermediate presence (2 to 7 percent) in South, Central, and Southwest Asia, Israel, Japan, eastern and southern Europe, Russia, areas around the Amazon River basin, Honduras, and Guatemala. Chronic HBV infection is high (at least 8 percent) in all of Africa, Southeast Asia (including China, Korea, Indonesia, and the Philippines), the Middle East (except Israel), South and Western Pacific islands, the interior Amazon River basin, and some parts of the Caribbean (Haiti and the Dominican Republic).

You and your child should know that the following situations can increase the risk of contracting hepatitis B when traveling in any of these areas:

- Any injury or illness that require invasive medical attention, such as an injection transfusion, stitches, or intravenous drip

- Dental work

- Sharing personal items, such as toothbrushes, drinking glasses, earrings

- Practices that perforate the skin, such as ear piercing, acupuncture, tattooing

- Unprotected sexual contact

The CDC recommends that all children and adolescents traveling to any area of the world with an intermediate to high risk of hepatitis B be vaccinated. Specifically:

- Infants and children should receive three doses of HBV vaccine before leaving the country.

- The interval between doses 2 and 3 should be a minimum of eight weeks; the interval between doses 1 and 3 should be at least sixteen weeks. The third dose should not be given before an infant is at least twenty-four weeks of age.

## How About Rabies?

Rabies virus is a type of viral encephalitis that is nearly always fatal unless the vaccine is given. The disease is caused by a virus introduced by a bite and saliva from an infected animal (e.g., bat, raccoon, fox, cat, dog, skunk). The virus attacks the central nervous system and causes anxiety, difficulty swallowing, and seizures. If you and your children are traveling in regions where exposure to street dogs and/or bats is possible, then rabies is a potential risk.

Even though fewer than ten people die of rabies each year in the United States, up to forty thousand Americans get the vaccine after they have had contact with animals. Rabies is a problem in densely populated areas of Africa and Asia, including India, where there are large populations of stray dogs. Between 30 and 60 percent of human rabies cases occur in children younger than 15 years old.

Avoidance is always the best approach when faced with the possibility of rabies. However, an alternative is a series of injections with a rabies vaccine. A preexposure immunization series consists of three injections, with the second injection given one week after the first, and the third given three to four weeks after the first. If your child is then exposed to rabies, two more injections will be necessary along with the rabies immune globulin. If your child has not been preimmunized and has been potentially exposed to rabies, a series of five rabies vaccine injections is necessary, with the second through fifth injections given three, seven, fourteen, and twenty-eight days after the first. Hopefully, your child will never have to experience these injections.

# GLOSSARY

**Acellular vaccine:** A vaccine that contains a part of the cellular material rather than complete cells.

**Active immunity:** The process by which the immune system produces antibodies against a specific disease. You can acquire active immunity in two ways: by vaccination or by contracting the disease. "Active immunity" usually refers to a lifetime of protection, although with vaccines several doses and boosters are sometimes needed to achieve this goal.

**Adjuvant:** A substance that is added during the production of a vaccine to boost the body's immune response to the vaccine. Adjuvants are also used when there is an insufficient supply of the antigen needed for the vaccine or when the antigen does not induce a good antibody response. Examples of adjuvants include albumin, aluminum salts, aluminum phosphate, and aluminum gels.

**Advisory Committee on Immunization Practices (ACIP):** A panel of ten experts composed of representatives from the Centers for Disease Control and Prevention, Food and Drug

Administration, National Institutes of Health, American Academy of Pediatrics, American Academy of Family Physicians, American Medical Association, and others, whose task is to make recommendations concerning the use of vaccines in the United States.

**Albumin:** A type of protein that is added to some vaccines as an excipient. Vaccines may contain one of three types of albumin: egg, human, or bovine (cow). Vaccines for both seasonal and H1N1 influenza typically contain egg albumin, while some vaccines for measles, mumps, and/or rubella contain human albumin.

**Allergy:** A condition in which the body reacts in an exaggerated way to a substance, such as pollen, a food, or a drug.

**Aluminum:** Aluminum salts, gels, and other forms are added as adjuvants to vaccines to stimulate a better immune response. Animal and human studies have shown that aluminum can cause the death of nerve cells, and it has been linked to memory loss, loss of concentration, and other brain injuries.

**Ammonium sulfate:** A substance registered as a pesticide adjuvant and used as a fertilizer. It is also added to some children's vaccines. Ammonium sulfate is a suspected toxicant of the gastrointestinal, respiratory, and nervous systems.

**Anaphylaxis:** A severe allergic reaction to a substance that typically occurs immediately after someone is exposed to the substance. Symptoms include breathing difficulties, loss of consciousness, and a serious drop in blood pressure.

**Antibiotics:** To prevent the growth of bacteria during vaccine production and storage, antibiotics are added to some vaccines. No vaccine made in the United States contains penicillin.

**Antibody:** A protein present in the blood that the body produces in response to invasion by foreign substances (antigens), such as viruses or bacteria. Antibodies protect the body from disease by attaching themselves to the foreign substances and destroying them.

**Antigens:** Foreign substances (e.g., bacteria, viruses, fungi) that are capable of causing disease. When antigens are present in the body, they can trigger an immune response, which typically is the production of antibodies. Antigens are used in vaccines to induce an immune response.

**Attenuated vaccine:** A vaccine in which a live virus is made weaker by subjecting it to chemical or physical processes so the weakened virus will trigger an immune response without causing severe effects of the disease. The attenuated childhood vaccines in the United States include those for measles, mumps, rubella, polio, yellow fever, and chicken pox (varicella). Attenuated vaccines are also referred to as live vaccines.

**Autism:** A developmental disorder that is characterized by significant problems with social interaction, communication difficulties, and repetitive behavior and interests. The cause of autism is not known, although several factors are likely involved, including genetics and environment.

**Bacteria:** Microorganisms, both beneficial and harmful, that are present throughout the environment. Some of those that can cause bacterial disease include ones for which vaccines have been developed; for example, diphtheria, tetanus, pneumococcal disease, and pertussis (whooping cough).

**Booster shots:** Additional doses of a vaccine given after one or more initial injections that are necessary to "boost" or enhance the immune system.

**Casamino acids:** A mixture of all the amino acids, except tryptophan, used as a growth medium.

**Combination vaccine:** A vaccine dose that contains two or more vaccines. An example is the MMR (measles/mumps/rubella) vaccine.

**Conjugated vaccine:** A vaccine that consists of two compounds joined together, typically a protein and a polysaccharide, which increases the vaccine's effectiveness.

**Endemic:** A term used to describe a disease that is present at a continual, low level within a community or region.

**Excipient:** An inactive substance that is used as a carrier for an active ingredient in a medication or supplement. An excipient can help the body better absorb an ingredient, or it can be used to increase the volume of formulations that contain potent active ingredients. Examples of excipients include binders, diluents, and preservatives.

**Febrile seizure:** A seizure that occurs as a result of a fever or unusually high body temperature. Approximately 4 percent of young children have at least one febrile seizure during their lifetime. Febrile seizures can occur with any common childhood illness that may cause fever. Most children recover quickly with no lasting side effects.

**Formaldehyde:** A toxic substance used to inactivate bacterial products used in toxoid vaccines (vaccines that use an inactive bacterial toxin to produce immunity), such as any of the tetanus, diphtheria, and pertussis vaccines. Formaldehyde is also added to destroy any unwanted bacteria and viruses that might contaminate the vaccine during production. Although most formaldehyde is removed from the vaccine before it is packaged, a minute amount remains in the final product.

**Formalin:** a 37 percent solution of formaldehyde in water, which is used for fixing and preserving biologic specimens for pathologic and histologic examination.

**Gelatin:** A substance derived from boiled pigs. (In foods, gelatins come from boiled cows.) Children who have severe allergies to gelatin should undergo skin testing before receiving a vaccine that contains gelatin.

**Glutaraldehyde:** A colorless liquid used to sterilized medical equipment and to treat industrial water and as a chemical preservative.

**Guillain-Barre syndrome:** A rare neurological disease in which individuals experience temporary paralysis and a loss of reflexes, as well as weakness, numbness, and increased sensitivity throughout the body. Symptoms usually begin over one day and may continue to worsen for three or four days up to three or four weeks. Most patients recover within two to four weeks once the progression stops, although the condition is fatal in 5 percent of cases.

**Immune globulin (also immunoglobulin):** A protein found in the blood that fights infection. Also known as gamma globulin, it is frequently administered immediately after exposure to an infection.

**Immune system:** A system in the body that is responsible for warding off and fighting disease. The immune system can identify foreign substances (e.g., bacteria, fungi, viruses, parasites) and develop a defense against them, known as the immune response. Initiation of the immune response involves the production of molecules called antibodies, which work to eliminate foreign organisms that invade the body.

**Immunity:** Protection against an infection or disease. There are two main types of immunity, passive and active. Immunity is determined by the presence of antibodies in the blood and is usually identified by a laboratory test.

**Immunization:** The process by which a person is protected against an infection or disease. The term "immunization" is often used interchangeably with "vaccination" and "inoculation."

**Immunosuppression:** A condition in which the immune system is not able to protect the body from infection and disease. Immunosuppression can be caused by certain drugs (e.g., chemotherapy drugs) and diseases that compromise the immune system, such as cancer and HIV. Anyone who has immunosuppression should not receive live, attenuated vaccines.

**Inactivated vaccine:** A vaccine that is prepared using viruses and bacteria that have been inactivated (killed) using either physical or chemical means. Inactivated organisms cannot cause disease.

**Incidence:** The number of new cases of disease reported in a specific population over a certain amount of time.

**Live vaccine:** A vaccine that uses a live virus weakened (attenuated) using chemical or physical means in order to produce an immune response without causing the effects of the disease. Live vaccines in the United States include those for measles, mumps, and rubella (MMR), varicella, and yellow fever.

**Monosodium glutamate (MSG):** A stabilizer used in a few vaccines to help the product remain unchanged when it is exposed to heat, acidity, humidity, or light. Some people are hypersensitive to MSG.

**Neomycin:** An antibiotic/antibacterial used in many children's vaccines. Children with a mild or moderate allergy to neomycin may experience a rash after receiving a vaccine that contains neomycin, while children with a severe allergy should avoid vaccines that contain this ingredient.

**Passive Immunity:** A state of being in which you are protected against infection or disease through antibodies produced by another human or animal. For example, a mother passes immunity to her child through the placenta. These antibodies protect the baby temporarily, typically for the first four to six months of life.

**Pathogens:** Organisms, such as viruses, bacteria, fungi, and parasites, that can cause infections and disease in humans.

**Phenol:** Phenol has anesthetic properties and is used in the production of vaccines and other drugs, weed killers, and synthetic resins.

**Polymyxin B:** An antibiotic/antibacterial used in some children's vaccines. Children with a mild or moderate allergy to polymyxin B may experience a rash after receiving a vaccine that contains polymyxin B, while children with a severe allergy should avoid vaccines that contain this ingredient.

**Polysaccharide vaccines:** Vaccines that are made of long chains of sugar molecules. Polysaccharide vaccines are available for *Haemophilus influenzae* type B, meningococcal disease, and pneumococcal disease.

**Polysorbate 80:** A detergent-type chemical that converts into sorbitol and ethylene oxide, which is more toxic than the original chemical, after it is injected into the body. Polysorbate 80 is used in pharmacology to help deliver certain drugs and other agents across the blood-brain barrier. Some experts worry that undesirable vaccine materials are transported across the blood-brain barrier with the help of polysorbate 80.

**Production media:** Materials in which vaccine components are cultured. Some of these media include bovine (cow) protein, chick embryo tissue, fertilized chicken eggs, human tissue, monkey kidney tissue, and yeast extract. Media are removed from the final product, but they are still present in trace amounts in the vaccine. These trace amounts may be problematic for some children who have allergies; for example, vaccines that use chicken embryo may cause an allergic reaction in children who are allergic to eggs.

**Recombinant:** A term referring to the result of a new combination of genetic materials or cells. Thus a recombinant vaccine is one that is the result of combining genetic materials from different sources.

**Sodium borate:** A neurotoxin that is not meant to be taken internally. However, it is found in some vaccines, including one for HPV. At a cellular level, sodium borate can cause changes to DNA. Symptoms include nausea, vomiting, diarrhea, seizures, shock, depression, hyperactivity, vascular collapse, and death.

**Sodium phosphate monobasic:** Also known as monohydrate, sodium biphosphate monohydrate, sodium acid phosphate monohydrate, and sodium dihydrogen phosphate monohydrate, an excipient that is slowly and incompletely absorbed when ingested.

**Strain:** A specific version of an organism.

**Suspending fluid:** Generally harmless substances (e.g., saline, sterile water, fluids that contain protein) used to deliver a vaccine, as in an injection.

**Thimerosal:** A mercury-containing preservative that is used in some vaccines. At one time, thimerosal was found in most vaccines, but concerns about possible mild to serious reactions to thimerosal led to the preservative being reduced or eliminated from vaccines as a precautionary measure. Currently only a few of the recommended childhood vaccines made for the U.S. vaccine market contain trace amounts of thimerosal.

**2-phenoxyethanol:** An alternative to thimerosal in vaccines, added to protect the product from changing when it is exposed to heat, acidity, humidity, or light. This ingredient is toxic and is also used as an insect repellent, a topical antiseptic, a solvent for dyes and inks, and in germicides. It is classed as very toxic.

**Vaccination:** Injection of weakened or killed infectious organisms designed to prevent disease.

**Vaccine:** A product that produces immunity and protects the body from disease. Vaccines are administered by injection, orally, or by aerosol, although the majority of vaccines for children are by injection.

**Vaccine Adverse Event Reporting System (VAERS):** A database for information and analysis of adverse events associated with vaccines currently licensed in the United States. VAERS is managed by the Centers for Disease Control and Prevention and the Food and Drug Administration.

# APPENDICES

## GETTING HELP WITH VACCINE COSTS

In today's world of high health-care costs, parents often worry about how much it will cost them to vaccinate their children. Parents who have health insurance usually, but not always, find that their policy covers baby immunizations recommended by the CDC and required to enroll their children in school. Some plans, however, do not cover childhood immunizations or only offer to pay for some of them.

That's why it is so important for you to consult your health insurance carrier to see how your plan handles childhood immunizations. If you discover your plan does not pay for one or more vaccines your child needs, you can ask your physician for a referral to a public clinic or where to get low-cost immunizations. (See "Vaccines for Children Program.")

According to a study published in the *Pediatrics* journal, parents whose infants are covered by health insurance can expect to pay $242 out of pocket for vaccinations during the first year of their child's life. Overall, immunizations for the first year cost at least $620 and the cost for all vaccinations needed during childhood and adolescence is now well more than $1,200 and climbing as more vaccines are added to the schedule, insurance plans change, and the costs of vaccines rise.

Not everyone can afford some or all childhood vaccinations. If you need some assistance providing the necessary vaccinations for your child, there are some free or low-cost options, which are discussed in this chapter.

## Vaccines for Children Program

If you are the parent or guardian of a child who needs vaccinations yet you cannot afford them, the Vaccines for Children (VFC) Program may be able to help. The Centers for Disease Control and Prevention administer the VFC Program, which helps provide vaccines to children who may not otherwise have access to them. The vaccines available through the VFC are for infants, young children, and adolescents and include all those recommended by the Advisory Committee on Immunization Practices and approved by the CDC.

The CDC buys and distributes the recommended vaccines to private and public health-care providers who are enrolled in the VFC Program. To be eligible for the VFC Program, a child must be younger than 19 years of age and meet one of the following requirements:

- Eligible for Medicaid

- Uninsured

- Underinsured, which means a child's health insurance does not cover vaccines, does not cover specific vaccines, or covers vaccines but has a fixed dollar limit for vaccines (if the latter is the case, once your child has reached that fixed dollar amount, he or she is eligible to receive free vaccines from the VFC Program)

- American Indian or Alaska Native

Free vaccines from the VFC Program are available only at Federally Qualified Health Centers (FQHCs) or Rural Health Clinics (RHCs). FQHCs must meet certain criteria under the Medicare and Medicaid programs. To locate an FQHC or RHC in your area, you should contact the VFC coordinator in your state. A list is provided on the CDC Web site: http://www.cdc.gov/vaccines/programs/vfc/contacts-state .htm. You can also call the CDC at 1-800-232-4636 and ask for the phone number of your state's VFC coordinator.

If your child is eligible for the VFC Program based on any of the preceding criteria, ask your doctor if he or she is a VFC Program provider. Approximately forty thousand doctors in the United States are enrolled in the VFC Program. If the answer is "no," then you can take your child to an FQHC, RHC, or public health clinic (contact your local health department) in your area.

Although there is no charge for any of the vaccines administered by a VFC provider to eligible children, parents may be faced with other costs associated with the vaccination itself. For example, doctors may charge a standard fee to administer each shot. If a family cannot afford to pay the per-shot fee, the physician must waive his or her fee. Therefore, no VFC-eligible child can be denied a vaccination because of his or her parent's or guardian's inability to afford the shot fee.

Doctors may also choose to charge for the office visit or for other services they deem necessary before the vaccine can be administered, such as an eye exam or a blood test. Parents should ask the office staff of the VFC provider they choose if these or other fees may be expected of them when they bring their child in for vaccination. These fees are not waived.

## Parents Beware: Not All Pediatricians Offer Vaccinations

Does your pediatrician or family doctor offer vaccinations for children? While this may sound like a ridiculous question, some doctors are backing out of the vaccine business, and the reason is cost.

A study published in the December 1, 2008, issue of *Pediatrics* reported that the high and continually rising costs of childhood vaccinations have led an increasing number of doctors to either stop providing vaccines or consider doing so to privately insured patients only. Five percent of pediatricians and 21 percent of family physicians surveyed said they had seriously considered not offering the vaccines recommended for infants and children.

A major reason for the doctors' dissatisfaction was the actual cost of the vaccines. At the time of the study, the cost of buying all the doses of the recommended pediatric vaccines had climbed from $600 per child in 2000 to $1,500 per child in 2008. Sixty-five percent of the polled physicians said they would not give a vaccine if the reimbursement amount was less than what it would cost them to purchase the vaccine.

A related study in the same issue of *Pediatrics* reported that 24 percent of practices polled had stopped giving vaccines to patients who had certain health plans or had discontinued their relationship with an insurance company because of inadequate reimbursement.

When shopping for a pediatrician, here are two more questions you should ask: "Do you give vaccinations?" If the answer is "yes," "which health plans or insurance companies do you accept?"


## CHILDREN'S VACCINATION SCHEDULES—2012

Please visit the following links to download the vaccination schedules for these age groups:

### CDC Vaccination Schedule for Children 0 to 6 Years

http://www.cdc.gov/vaccines/recs/schedules/downloads/child/0-6yrs-schedule-bw.pdf

## CDC Vaccination Schedule for Children 7 to 18 Years

http://www.cdc.gov/vaccines/recs/schedules/downloads
/child/7-18yrs-schedule-bw.pdf

## Catch-up Vaccination Schedule

http://www.cdc.gov/vaccines/recs/schedules/downloads
/child/catchup-schedule-bw.pdf

# RESOURCES

## American Academy of Pediatrics

http://www.aap.org/

This Web site by the AAP provides information on immunizations, childhood diseases, and more.

## American College for Advancement in Medicine (ACAM)

http://www.acamnet.org/site/c.ltJWJ4MPIwE/b.5420171/k
.76F0/Integrative_Medicine_From_ACAM__the_voice_of
_integrative_medicine.htm

This ACAM Web site offers individuals an opportunity to search for MDs and DOs who practice integrative medicine in their area.

## American Holistic Medical Association

http://www.holisticmedicine.org/

This Web site offers individuals an opportunity to locate a holistic, integrative physician in their area.

## History of Vaccines, The

http://www.historyofvaccines.org/content/timelines/diseases-and-vaccines

This Web site provides a history of vaccines; it is a project of the College of Physicians of Philadelphia.

## Holistic Pediatric Association

http://hpakids.org/

This Web site helps parents make informed choices on behalf of their children, based on a holistic model of health care.

## Immunization Action Coalition: State Mandates on Immunization and Vaccine-Preventable Diseases

http://www.immunize.org/laws/

This Web site offers access to lists of which immunizations are required by each of the fifty states plus Washington, D.C., for entry into school.

## Institute for Vaccine Safety

http://www.vaccinesafety.edu/

A Web site by the Johns Hopkins Bloomberg School of Public Health, it provides an independent assessment of vaccines and vaccine safety for the general public, physicians, and decision makers.

## National Vaccine Information Center

http://www.nvic.org/

This is the Web site for a national charitable, nonprofit educational organization advocating for vaccine safety and informed consent protections.

## ThinkTwice Global Vaccine Network

http://www.thinktwice.com/

This Web site offers "an extensive selection of uncensored information on childhood shots and other immunizations."

## Vaccine Excipient & Media Summary: Excipients Included in U.S. Vaccines, by Vaccine

http://www.cdc.gov/vaccines/pubs/pinkbook/downloads /appendices/B/excipient-table-2.pdf

This Web site lists the excipients found and media culture used in the production of U.S.-licensed vaccines.

## World Association for Vaccine Education (WAVE)

http://www.novaccine.com/

This Web site is comprehensive resource for information on vaccine ingredients.

# ENDNOTES

## INTRODUCTION

F. Zhou et al., "Economic Evaluation of Routine Childhood Immunization with DTaP, Hib, IPV, MMR, and Hep B Vaccines in the United States," Pediatric Academic Societies Conference, Seattle, Washington, May 2003.

Bill & Melinda Gates Foundation press release, http://www.gatesfoundation.org/press-releases/Pages/decade-of-vaccines-wec-announcement-100129.aspx.

Katherine Dettwyler, PhD, "The Natural Age of Weaning," http://www.whale.to/a/dettwyler.html.

## CHAPTER 1

http://www.historyofvaccines.org/content/timelines/smallpox.

E Leuridan et al., "Kinetics of Maternal Antibodies Against

Rubella and Varicella in Infants," *Vaccine* 29(11) (March 3, 2011): 2222–26.


## CHAPTER 2

C. S. Price et al., "Prenatal and Infant Exposure to Thimerosal from Vaccines and Immunoglobins and Risk of Autism," *Pediatrics*; 126(4) (October 2010): 656–64.

American Academy of Pediatrics, "Aluminum Toxicity in Infants and Children," *Pediatrics*; 97 (1996):413–16.

Centers for Disease Control and Prevention, "Vaccine Excipient & Media Summary: Excipients Included in U.S. Vaccines, by Vaccine," http://www.cdc.gov/vaccines/pubs/pinkbook/downloads/appendices/B/excipient-table-2.pdf.

Centers for Disease Control and Prevention, http://www.cdc.gov/vaccines/vac-gen/additives.htm.

S. L. Deeks et al., "An Assessment of Mumps Vaccine Effectiveness by Dose During an Outbreak in Canada," May 16, 2011, doi: 10.1503/cmaj.101371.

B. Deer, "How the Case Against the MMR Vaccine Was Fixed," *British Medical Journal* 342 (January 5, 2011): c5347.

Editors, "Retraction—Ileal-Lymphoid-Nodular Hyperplasia, Non-specific Colitis, and Pervasive Developmental Disorder in Children, *The Lancet* 375(9713) (February 6, 2010): 445.

Boyd Haley to the Honorable Dan Burton, Chairman of the Committee on Government Reform, http://www.whale.to/m/haley.html.

Institute for Vaccine Safety, http://www.vaccinesafety.edu/components-Excipients.htm.

A. Kennedy et al., "Confidence About Vaccines in the United States: Understanding Parents' Perceptions," *Health Affairs* 30(6) (June 2011): 1151–59.

Lawrence B. Palevsky, "Aluminum and Vaccine Ingredients: What Do We Know? What Don't We Know?" http://www.nvic.org/Doctors-Corner/Aluminum-and-Vaccine-Ingredients.aspx.

C. A. Shaw et al., "Aluminum Hydroxide Injections Lead to Motor Deficits and Motor Neuron Degeneration," *Journal of Inorganic Biochemistry*, 103(11) (Nov. 2009): 1555.

G. Stohr, "Suits Against Vaccine Makers Curbed by U.S. Supreme Court," February 22, 2011, http://www.bloomberg.com/news/2011-02-22/suits-against-vaccine-makers-curbed-by-u-s-supreme-court-in-pfizer-case.html.

## CHAPTER 3

Hepatitis B Foundation, http://www.hepb.org/professionals/approved_brands.htm and http://www.hepb.org/hepb/statistics.htm.

American Congress of Obstetricians and Gynecologists, http://www.acog.org/publications/patient_education/bp093.cfm.

Centers for Disease Control and Prevention, http://www.cdc.gov/hepatitis/ChooseB.htm.

Centers for Disease Control and Prevention, http://www.cdc.gov/vaccines/vac-gen/side-effects.htm.

J. B. Classen, "Childhood Immunization and Diabetes Mellitus," *New Zealand Medical Journal* 109(1022) (May 24, 1996): 195.

C. M. Gallagher and M. S. Goodman, "Hepatitis B Vaccination of Male Neonates and Autism Diagnosis, NHIS 1997–2002," *Journal of Toxicology and Environmental Health A* 73(24) (2010): 1665–77.

D. A. Geier and M. R. Geier, "A Case-Control Study of Serious Autoimmune Adverse Events Following Hepatitis B Immunization," *Autoimmunity* 38(4) (June 2005): 295–301.

D. A. Geier, "Chronic Adverse Reactions Associated with Hepatitis B Vaccination," *Annals of Pharmacotherapy* 36 (12) (2002): 1970–71.

M. A. Hernan et al., "Recombinant Hepatitis B Vaccine and the Risk of Multiple Sclerosis: A Prospective Study," *Neurology* 63(5) (September 14, 2004): 838–42.

Immunization Action Coalition, http://www.vaccineinformation.org/hepb/.

Infectious Diseases Society of America, Abstract 814, "Risk Factors for Non-Receipt of Hepatitis B Vaccine in the Newborn Nursery," accessed June 26, 2011, http://idsa.confex.com/idsa/2010/webprogram/Paper3284.html.

Y. Mikaeloff et al., "Hepatitis B Vaccine and the Risk of CNS Inflammatory Demyelination in Childhood," *Neurology* 72(10) (March 10, 2009): 873–80.

H. Petousis-Harris and N. Turner, "Hepatitis B Vaccination and Diabetes," *New Zealand Medical Journal* 112(1093) (August 13, 1999): 303–4.

Paolo Pozzilli, MD, from WebMD: http://www.rense.com /general2/vacin.htm.

Jane Orient, M.D., Statement of the Association of American Physicians & Surgeons to the Subcommittee on Criminal Justice, Drug Policy, and Human Resources of the Committee on Government Reform, U.S. House of Representatives, http://articles.mercola.com/sites/articles/archive /2008/01/02/hepatitis-b-vaccine-part-four.aspx.


## CHAPTER 4


FDA on rotavirus vaccines, http://www.fda.gov/News Events/PublicHealthFocus/ucm205585.htm.

National Network for Immunization Information, http:// www.immunizationinfo.org/vaccines/rotavirus#toc-top.

Centers for Disease Control and Prevention, "Prevention of Rotavirus Gastroenteritis Among Infants and Children: Recommendations of the Advisory Committee on Immunization Practices (ACIP)," MMWR,55(RR12) (August 11, 2006): 1–13.

Centers for Disease Control and Prevention, "ACIP Provisional Recommendations for the Prevention of Rotavirus Gastroenteritis Among Infants and Children," http://www.cdc .gov/vaccines/recs/provisional/downloads/roto-7-1-08.pdf.

Centers for Disease Control and Prevention, "Rotarix Rotavirus Vaccine: Rare Side Effect Possible," September 2010, http://www.cdc.gov/vaccines/vpd-vac/rotavirus/Vac-label -parents.htm.

Food and Drug Administration, Update of Recommendations for the Use of Rotavirus Vaccines, 2010. http://www

.fda.gov/BiologicsBloodVaccines/Vaccines/ApprovedProd
ucts/ucm212140.htm

"GlaxoSmithKline Product Information," https://www
.gsksource.com/gskprm/en/US/adirect/gskprm?cmd=Product
DetailPage&product_id=1244173585205&featureKey
=600594.

Institute for Vaccine Safety package inserts, http://www
.vaccinesafety.edu/package_inserts.htm.

S. Lee et al., "Development of a Bacillus Subtilis-Based
Rotavirus Vaccine," *Clinical and Vaccine Immunology*
17(11) (2010): 1647–55.

"Merck & Co. Product Information," http://www.merck
.com/product/usa/pi_circulars/r/rotateq/rotateq_ppi.pdf.

U. Parashar et al., "Rotavirus and Severe Childhood
Diarrhea," *Emerging Infectious Diseases* 12(2) (2006):
304–06.

## CHAPTER 5

The Children's Hospital of Philadelphia, http://www.chop
.edu/service/vaccine-education-center/a-look-at-each-vaccine
/dtap-diphtheria-tetanus-and-pertussis-vaccine.html.

Institute for Vaccine Safety, Johns Hopkins Bloomberg
School of Public Health, http://www.vaccinesafety.edu/com
ponents-DTaP.htm.

National Network for Immunization Information, http://
www.immunizationinfo.org/vaccines/tetanus.

## CHAPTER 6

M. C. Thigpen et al., "Bacterial Meningitis in the United States, 1998–2007," *New England Journal of Medicine* 364 (May 26, 2011): 2016–25.

Centers for Disease Control and Prevention, http://www.cdc.gov/vaccines/vpd-vac/hib/ (package insert information)

Centers for Disease Control and Prevention, "*Haemophilus influenzae* Type B," in W. Atkinson et al., eds., *Epidemiology and Prevention of Vaccine-Preventable Diseases,* 11th ed. (Washington, DC: Public Health Foundation. 2009), pp. 71–84.

Food and Drug Administration, http://www.fda.gov/downloads/BiologicsBloodVaccines/Vaccines/ApprovedProducts/UCM109841.pdf.

Immunization Action Coalition, http://www.vaccineinformation.org/hib/qandadis.asp.

National Network for Immunization Information, http://www.immunizationinfo.org/vaccines/haemophilus-influenzae-type-b-hib.

Bob Sears, http://www.askdrsears.com/default.asp.

## CHAPTER 7

R. Rappuoli, et al., "Vaccine Discovery and Translation of New Vaccine Technology," *Lancet*, June 9, 2011.

R. Andrews and S. A. Moberley, "The Controversy over the Efficacy of Pneumococcal Vaccine," *Canadian Medical Association Journal* 180 (2009): 18–19.

M. T. Dransfield et al., "Superior Immune Response to Protein-Conjugate Versus Free Pneumococcal Polysaccharide Vaccine in Chronic Obstructive Pulmonary Disease," *American Journal of Respiratory and Critical Care Medicine* 180 (2009): 499–505.

A. Huss et al., "Efficacy of Pneumococcal Vaccination in Adults: A meta-analysis," *Canadian Medical Association Journal* 180 (2009): 48–58.

J. Johnstone, "Review: Pneumococcal Vaccination Is Not Effective for Preventing Pneumonia, Bacteraemia, Bronchitis, or Mortality," *Evidence-Based Medicine* 14 (2009): 109.

T. Maruyama et al., "Efficacy of 23-Valent Pneumococcal Vaccine in Preventing Pneumonia and Improving Survival in Nursing Home Residents: Double Blind, Randomised and Placebo Controlled Trial," *British Medical Journal* 340 (2010): c1004.

S. A. Moberley et al., "Vaccines for Preventing Pneumococcal Infection in Adults (Cochrane Review), in *The Cochrane Library* (Chichester, UK: Wiley)

National Foundation for Infectious Diseases, http://www .nfid.org/factsheets/pneumofacts.shtml.

J. P. Nuorti and C. G. Whitney, "Prevention of Pneumococcal Disease Among Infants and Children—Use of 13-Valent Pneumococcal Conjugate Vaccine and 23-Valent Pneumococcal Polysaccharide Vaccine. Recommendations and Reports," *Morbidity and Mortality Weekly Report* 59 (RR11) (December 10, 2010): 1–18, http://www.cdc.gov/mmwr/preview/mmwrhtml/rr5911a1.htm?s_cid=rr5911a1_w.

"Pfizer Product Information for Prevnar and Prevnar-13," http://labeling.pfizer.com/showlabeling.aspx?id=134 and http://labeling.pfizer.com/ShowLabeling.aspx?id=501.

Pfizer Medical Customer Service: 800-438-1985, calls in April and May 2011.

W. Zhou et al., "Surveillance for Safety After Immunization: Vaccine Adverse Event Reporting System (VAERS)—United States, 1991–2001," *Morbidity and Mortality Weekly Report* 52(SS-1) (2003).

## CHAPTER 8

Lawrence K. Altman, "Panel Advises Flu Shots for Children up to Age 18, *New York Times,* February 28, 2008, http://www.nytimes.com/2008/02/28/health/28flu.html.

"Update: Recommendations of the Advisory Committee on Immunization Practices (ACIP) Regarding Use of CSL Seasonal Influenza Vaccine (Afluria) in the United States During 2010–11," *Morbidity and Mortality Weekly Report* 59(31) (August 13, 2010): 989–992.

National Network for Immunization Information, http://www.immunizationinfo.org/vaccines/influenza.

## CHAPTER 9

S. L. Deeks et al., "An Assessment of Mumps Vaccine Effectiveness By Dose During an Outbreak in Canada," *Canadian Medical Association Journal* 183 (9) (June 14, 2011): 1014–20

National Network for Immunization Information, http://www.immunizationinfo.org/vaccines/measles.

"Mumps," http://kidshealth.org/parent/infections/bacterial_viral/mumps.html.

H. V. Ratajczak, "Theoretical Aspects of Autism: Causes—a

review," http://www.rescuepost.com/files/theoretical-aspects-of-autism-causes-a-review1-1.pdf.


# CHAPTER 10

Centers for Disease Control and Prevention, http://www.cdc.gov/vaccines/vpd-vac/combo-vaccines/mmrv/vacopt-factsheet-parent.htm.

WebMD, http://children.webmd.com/vaccines/news/20110602/vaccination-rate-for-kids-is-over-90-percent.


# CHAPTER 11

U.S. Global Health Policy, http://globalhealth.kff.org/Daily-Reports/2011/May/19/GH051911-WHO-Reform.aspx.

http://www.nlm.nih.gov/medlineplus/ency/article/002030.htm.

J. P. Alexander et al., "Transmission of Imported Vaccine-Derived Poliovirus in an Undervaccinated Community in Minnesota," *Journal of Infectious Diseases* 199(3) (February 1, 2009): 391–97.


# CHAPTER 12

D. Daniels et al., "Surveillance for Acute Viral Hepatitis—United States, 2007," *Morbidity and Mortality Weekly Report Surveillance Summary* 58 (SS03) (May 22, 2009): 1–27.

National Institutes of Health, http://www.ncbi.nlm.nih.gov/pubmedhealth/PMH0001323/.

K. Sweet et al., "Hepatitis A Infection in Recent International Adoptees and Their Contacts in Minnesota, 2007–2009," *Pediatrics* 128(2) (July 4, 2011), online.

## CHAPTER 13

L. H. Harrison et al., "Risk Factors for Meningococcal Disease in Students in Grades 9–12," *Pediatric Infectious Disease Journal* 27(3) (March 2008): 193–99.

"Menveo PI," https://www.novartisvaccinesdirect.com/PDF/Menveo_Full_Promotional_PI.pdf.

Mercury News, http://www.mercurynews.com/breaking-news/ci_17884705?nclick_check=1.

Novartis, http://www.novartisvaccines.com/products-diseases/meningitis-vaccines/meningitis-vaccines.shtml.

Society for Adolescent Health and Medicine/Internal Medicine News, http://www.internalmedicinenews.com/news/adolescent-medicine/single-article/uptake-of-meningococcal-vaccine-awareness-is-not-enough/95e25c7471.html.

J. Tully et al., "Risk and Protective Factors for Meningococcal Disease in Adolescents: Matched Cohort Study," *British Medical Journal* 332(7539) (February 25, 2006): 445–50

## CHAPTER 14

J. M. L. Brotherton et al., "Early Effect of the HPV Vaccination Programme on Cervical Abnormalities in Victoria, Australia: An Ecological Study," *The Lancet* 377 (9783) (2011): 2085–92.

Centers for Disease Control and Prevention, http://www.cdc.gov/vaccinesafety/vaccines/hpv/gardasil.html.

Charlotte Haug, MD, PhD, MSc, "The Risks and Benefits of HPV Vaccination," *JAMA* 302(7) (2009): 795–96.

NIH, National Institute of Allergy and Infectious Diseases.

B. A. Slade et al., "Postlicensure Safety Surveillance for Quadrivalent Human Papillomavirus Recombinant Vaccine," *JAMA* 302(7) (August 19, 2009): 750–57.


## CHAPTER 15

A. Kempe et al., "Prevalence of Parental Concerns About Childhood Vaccines: The Experience of Primary Care Physicians," *American Journal of Preventive Medicine* 40(5) (May 2011): 548–55.

R. W. Sears, MD, FAAP, *The Vaccine Book: Making the Right Decision for Your Child.* New York: Little, Brown and Company, 2007.

Kenneth Bock, M.D., *Healing the New Childhood Epidemics: Autism, ADHD, Asthma, and Allergies: The Groundbreaking Program for the 4-A Disorders* (New York: Ballantine, 2008).

D. R. Feikin et al., "Individual and Community Risks of Measles and Pertussis Associated with Personal Exemptions to Immunization," *JAMA* 282 (2000): 3145–50.

E. A. Flanagan-Klygis et al., "Dismissing the Family Who Refuses Vaccines: A Study of Pediatrician Attitudes," *Archives of Pediatrics & Adolescent Medicine* 159(10) (October 2005): 929–34.

K. M. Malone and A. R. Hinman, "Vaccination Mandates: The Public Health Imperative and Individual Rights," in

R. A. Goodman, et al., eds., *Law in Public Health Practice* (New York: Oxford University Press, 2003), pp. 262–284.

"Measles—United States, January 1–April 25, 2008," *Mortality and Morbidity Weekly Report* 57 (2008): 494–98.

Donald W. Miller, MD, "A User Friendly Vaccination Schedule," http://www.safbaby.com/an-alternative-vaccina tion-schedule-from-dr-donald-miller.

National Vaccine Information Center, http://www.nvic.org /vaccine-laws.aspx.

Vaccine Ethics.org, http://www.vaccineethics.org/issue _briefs/industry.php

Offit study source, http://www.sciencedaily.com/releases /2002/01/020109073542.htm.

S. B. Omer et al., "Nonmedical Exemptions to School Immunization Requirements: Secular Trends and Association of State Policies with Pertussis Incidence," *JAMA* 296 (2006): 1757–63.

WHO, http://www.immunize.org/concerns/porcine.pdf.

## CHAPTER 16

Centers for Disease Control and Prevention, http://www.cdc .gov/ncidod/dvbid/yellowfever/YF_FactSheet.html.

Centers for Disease Control and Prevention, http://wwwnc .cdc.gov/travel/.

National Network for Immunization Information, http:// www.immunizationinfo.org/vaccines/rabies.

# APPENDICES

Cost Helper, http://www.costhelper.com/cost/child/baby -immunization.html.

G. L. Freed et al., "Primary Care Physician Perspective on Reimbursement for Childhood Immunizations," *Pediatrics* 122(6) (December 1, 2008): 1319–24.

G. L. Freed et al., "Variation in Provider Vaccine Purchase Prices and Payer Reimbursement," *Pediatrics* 122(6) (December 1, 2008a): 1325–31.

N. A. M. Molinari et al., "Out-of-pocket Costs of Childhood Immunizations: A Comparison by Type of Insurance Plan," *Pediatrics* 120(5) (November 2007): 1148–56.